th Asperger's

My Life
With Asperger's

Megan Hammond

NEW HOLLAND

First published in Australia in 2010 by
New Holland Publishers (Australia) Pty Ltd
Sydney • Auckland • London • Cape Town
www.newholland.com.au
1/66 Gibbes Street Chatswood NSW 2067 Australia
218 Lake Road Northcote Auckland New Zealand
86 Edgware Road London W2 2EA United Kingdom
80 McKenzie Street Cape Town 8001 South Africa
Copyright © 2010 in text: Megan Hammond
Copyright © 2010 in images: Gordon Hammond
Copyright © 2010 New Holland Publishers (Australia) Pty Ltd
Reprinted 2010

Author's note: The names of some individuals have been changed.

National Library of Australia Cataloguing-in-Publication entry
Hammond, Megan.
Living with Asperger's / Megan Hammond.
1st ed.
ISBN: 9781741107883 (pbk.)
Asperger's syndrome--Popular works.
616.8588

Publisher: Fiona Schultz
Publishing manager: Lliane Clarke
Project editor: Helen McGarry
Proofreader: Nina Paine
Designer: Amanda Tarlau
Production manager: Olga Dementiev
Printer: McPherson's Printing Group, Victoria

Dedication

I dedicate this book to my whole family who have stuck by me,
also
to all the ladies in the writing group for their belief in me.

Acknowledgements

Firstly I would like to thank my long-suffering parents, my brother Cameron, and my extended family for sticking by me through thick and thin!

Secondly I would like to thank Gaby Mason who teaches the writing course and group that I still attend, for her support. An extremely big thank you goes to all the patient, wise, caring, wonderful, understanding, supportive women who have attended the group over the years including Caroline, Paula, Louise, Carole, Agnes, Faye, Helen and Ruth.

I'd also like to thank Christine Paul, who was my teacher for the first writing course I had ever been to in my life. A thank you goes to another writing course run through the Manly Community College as well.

I would like to thank all my church and Bible study friends who have been there every step of the way along this road. I appreciate all their unconditional love, understanding and support, which have made me a better person.

I also would like to thank my other friends Jackie, Justine and Beck who have taught me different things when going out to places.

A big thank you goes to Dr Milch who has been there for me over the past 10 years or so when I've needed help from him. Thanks also to all the staff at the clinics I've been to for accepting me in extremely bad emotional states. They should be remembered more ...

Another thank you goes to all the professionals who have seen me over the years and their dedication to trying to find out what was wrong with me. We all know the mystery has been solved!

A special thanks to my patient and careful editors, Helen McGarry and Jenny Scepanovic. Their advice and understanding have been invaluable.

Contents

Foreword   10

This Is Me: Aspie Girl   13

1.   A Terrible Tuesday To Remember   15
2.   The Mystery Years   19
3.   Primary School Daze— An Educational Fog   23
4.   High School Hiccups   31
5.   Juggling Jobs   43
6.   Not Another Doc! Finally, A Diagnosis   53
7.   It's Not All Bad—Asperger's Symptoms And Strengths   60
8.   How Asperger's Has Affected Me   73
9.   Finding—And Losing—Love   94
10. Falling Through The Cracks—And Finding My Feet   107
11. Tricks Of The Trade—How I've Learned To Cope   120
12. Living As An Adult With Asperger's   129
13. Coming Out Of The Asperger's Fog   137
14. Notes From Megan's Family   140

Appendix   156

FOREWORD

As Megan's treating psychiatrist, it is an honour to have been invited to write this foreword.

Megan's experience of Asperger's disorder is at the core of this book. This developmental disorder is diagnosed when there are deficits in social relatedness, communication skills and restricted areas of interest. This is commonly associated with emotional vulnerability and learning difficulties. It is one of the more common autistic spectrum disorders. Autism had previously been identified in one in every 1000 individuals. More recently autistic spectrum disorders have been recognised in one in every 100 people. This is thus relevant to the world we live in today.

Megan's developmental experience has shifted on her journey from survival towards competence. To my mind, the production of this book is a milestone in this regard.

Megan has shared with us her very personal journey.

She describes how helpful it can be to find a label, a diagnosis, a way of making sense of her particular experience. As a professional, it is all too easy to focus on diagnostic and clinical issues. As a member of the general public, it can be hard to get your head around what this is all about. As a consumer, Megan has given us a glimpse of what this means for the individual.

Writing and other forms of self-expression offer a pathway for working through one's experiences. It has been exciting to share with Megan her motivation and purpose in the preparation of this book. Structure and deadlines are all a part of the ride. Creativity provides such an important outlet, an avenue to explore meaning.

Megan has shared her pain. Her confusion has been a source of profound distress, particularly within the domain of relationships. Her openness should be treated with respect. It is distressing that so often it is greeted with misunderstanding.

The following pages will add to the reader's insight, tolerance and respect for those who experience developmental challenges. Megan's writing is both generous and courageous. The journey is one that is all too human, one that will touch us all.

Antony Milch
MBBS FRANZCP Cert Ch Psych

This Is Me: Aspie Girl

I am not an animal! Nor am I retarded or even brain damaged! I am not someone else's project! I have very real and human emotions. I'm not unlike you.

It's just that sometimes for me things are scarier to deal with because I haven't got people-intuition. My world is ordered with routines while the outside world around me is powered by massive change and chaos. I am not blind to what's going on around me, yet I see things with often a very different slant or perspective.

I can hear a multitude of words and can take them very literally. Like the other night I heard, 'We're ladies and we're allowed to wag or flap our gums!'

It means talking, as I worked out, yet I was taking it literally, trying to do the expression for gums wagging. I must have looked a sight to the group of people I was sitting at a table with, but they didn't say anything to me. Luckily.

I love the sound, repetition, diversity and sameness of language because you can experiment with it and play with the different sounds. Sometimes I hear different words or sayings or things and I repeat them over to myself a few times. To feel words rolling off your tongue producing sound is amazing for me. Words are like raindrops soaking me with much needed information. But sometimes I get so confused with the different actions and reactions of people around me. Their 'doublespeak' reminds me of the book 1984 in which information is twisted beyond comprehension.

Speech for me has always been extremely confronting because I don't speak properly or clearly—even as an adult. I slur my words and talk reasonably slowly with a monotone that has no real expression or body to it.

Over the years, the drone has been a real drain for me as my confidence has gurgled downwards. Sometimes I became almost mute and asked others to do the speaking for me. It got to the point where my school friends would go up and ask for assorted lollies for me from the jars in the newsagency at the bus stop before school. They also helped find out things I wanted to know from the teachers.

Writing small notes and passing them to others in the class was useful for me because I didn't want to speak. Unfortunately the teachers didn't see it that way. I kept getting into trouble for passing notes in class. A few of them were intercepted by the wrong people who read them and then started hassling me even more as a result of it.

It didn't matter what I said or did because nobody ever really cared, listened to me or understood what I was feeling. Life was magic ... NOT!

I literally hated the sound of my own voice and wished many a time that I was mute, living in a world of silence. For me the silence was a whole lot safer as I didn't have to try to explain things.

Yet I could lose myself in the immense noise of heavy metal music and the quietness of writing poetry where I felt almost normal. I gave up the will to try to explain and express myself when nobody seemed to listen anyway. After all, the many, many doctors and specialists I'd been to over my lifetime had heard what I said and yet there were still an eternity of questions with no useful answers for me.

To waste emotional effort on talking wasn't worth it with people who didn't 'get' or understand me.

This book is to help others to understand what it is to have Asperger's syndrome. Through writing this book I believe I have finally found my voice.

1

A Terrible Tuesday To Remember

Suddenly I wake with a snippet of a memory. I have no idea where I am! Bursting through a bubble of consciousness my reality is absolute agony. I feel so unloved.

Around me TAFE teachers and staff are buzzing in a frenzy. Where am I? I seem to be in some type of office or reception area. Slowly my eyes shut again and I vaguely remember a stretcher.

'Oh my crumbs! Have I succeeded? Have I died? Am I actually in heaven? What's going on?' Everything is hazy. Then I'm swept into nothingness again. Something uncomfortable is choking me, going down my throat … then I feel a painful prick in my arm.

I haven't died because the pain is still coming fast. Cold sheets are stretched against my skin and a hospital smell sears up my nostrils.

I am 18 and I can see no future. I so much want to be dead and off this small Earth.

~

Throughout the rest of the day I was in a drug stupor, my memory fragmented, which was probably best for me. I remember suddenly waking. In my dreamlike state I saw both my parents looking stunned.

I couldn't bear the sight of them being there. My mouth was so dry and I wiped my hand over it only to find black stuff on my fingers. I discovered later that it was charcoal to suck up the poisons in my system. Yet within myself I felt so toxic and worthless anyway! For the life of me I couldn't work out what was happening. I wanted a drink of water.

Later that night I needed to go to the toilet but was too weak to get up, so the nursing staff got me a bedpan. Being helped up and held while doing so was so embarrassing. I wasn't a kid. I was an adult!

One of the last things I remember was sitting in the back of the classroom swallowing tablets—and more tablets, and then some more tablets—because I wanted the pain to go away. It had been building up for many months. No-one in class had noticed. Not the pain, or my solution to it.

I was studying Office Administration at TAFE, but it seemed I was back in school again. I felt so alone with myself and so sick of life in all ways. I didn't care for tomorrow.

Later I was told that I had walked to the shopping mall where one of my teachers found me, then brought me back to TAFE.

Suddenly I remembered that it was my brother Cameron's 16th birthday. Did I get him a present or a card, I asked myself? Then like a shot to the head I remembered I had written him a 'goodbye letter' for his birthday. Some present!

I drifted into a dreamless sleep where memories ceased to exist. Next day I was visited by a doctor asking me all kinds of questions that I didn't understand. I was surprised that breath was still passing through my body.

Over the next few days I slept like a tranquillised animal. No wonder, as I had overdosed on 70 tablets or more—a couple of handfuls of Valium, Restavits and other muscle relaxants. The effects of the drugs in my system stayed with me for 10 days or more. My head swam with what had happened and my body followed it. Through the fog I couldn't believe that I was still alive after what I had done to myself. My hope was for the comfort and peace of death, yet that wasn't to be!

Over the next few weeks, coming to terms with what had happened was hard for the whole family. For a long time my mother could not say 'suicide attempt'. She called it 'when you got sick'. I hated that. It was a suicide attempt and I had really wanted to die and have it all over.

Yet little did I know that another life-changing event was going to happen to me just one month later on Sunday, 5 May 1991. I fell in love for the first time and boy, was I so glad to be alive then!

A story or book starts with one word—here is mine:

IF ...

If my life ended that day ...
What would have been different?
Everything, is the case
I would've stopped ...
Right there and then ...
On that hospital bed
Aged just 18 years
With a whole life ahead
A future to be lived
A family torn apart
Right at the very seams
Devastation everywhere
For everyone involved
A tragedy never to get over
A young life wasted
And for what?
Nothing in the long run ...
I don't think ...
Just another number on a statistic list
Another casualty of society
Yet someone was watching over
Every single one of us that day
Protecting and guarding
Over this 'What if?' scenario

And for whatever reasons...
Things were different
And I came out living
Rising as a phoenix from the flames
Going into an unknown future ...
With quite a bit of it now known
Shared with smiles, laughter, adventure and tears
Meeting many different people, friends and family
Moulding to what I am today
Entirely with God's help
There are many 'What ifs' in life
We'll never understand
Yet I know only one thing ...
We all have one life to live
The best way we can
In this beautiful ...
Big wide world of ours!

© Megan Hammond, 2006

2

The Mystery Years

Western Australia, 1974 onwards

'Jesus! Jesus! I want to be Jesus! I want to be Jesus on the cross!' My three-year-old voice came out of my chest with so much passion to whoever could hear me.

My young brother just looked up at me, and then took his attention back to whatever he was doing. Running and skipping across the yard I grabbed pieces of wood, placing them carefully on the lawn. I then hurriedly stripped off to my undies lying on my own makeshift cross, absolutely proud of myself!

'I'm Jesus! I'm just like Jesus on the cross, mum!' I told her as she walked out the back door.

She didn't look too impressed but I think she went along with it. I was a really radical Christian extremist doing whatever I could think of at the time.

When we went overseas around my fourth birthday, I was worse. The instant we hit Italy it was, 'MUM! Can I have a crucifix please? Can I have Jesus on the cross please, please, plleeaaase!'

All through Italy those questions came up and I had no idea why I wasn't allowed to have any pictures of Saint Mary and all the others. My dad was a pastor of the Seventh-day Adventist Church and it would have looked strange with me, his daughter, coming back with Catholic paraphernalia. My parents decided I was a closet Catholic, nicknaming me 'Sister Mary Megan' for fun.

I was so obsessed with crosses and religious symbols like that for ages. Actually I am still interested in them and have a small collection.

When we visited Rome we entered a very small, little-known church and I was absolutely fascinated with it because death was a mystery to me too. All you could see from wall to wall were skeletons and bones of hundreds of dead monks everywhere. Wherever you looked there was a bone, skull or another fragment of what was once a monk. I stood in absolute awe of all this when most kids would be running off screaming and crying.

I wanted to know more and why they were all like that in the church. To keep me quiet my parents bought me a couple of postcards to look at when we got back home, even though my morbid fascination seemed strange to them at the time.

Upon reaching Israel, which was stinking hot at the time, I became a real task for my parents. They'd brought summer outfits for all of us, to keep ourselves cool. At the time I strongly disliked anything sleeveless such as dresses, singlets or anything like that which didn't cover my shoulders.

As we passed through the markets everyone was fascinated by my brother's extremely fair blond hair and gave us little presents. Meanwhile I was traipsing all around the place continually trying to pull my straps down in a vain attempt to cover my shoulders, with a sour look on my face. I hated it for some obscure reason all of my own!

People tell me I was an intelligent, quiet little kid and was always attracted to books and music. I had the most amazing memory, even helping my parents sometimes with different tasks. Quite often they would misplace things and then they would ask me if I had seen it and knew where it was. I'd go off and shuffle around for a bit and then come back with whatever they were looking for at the time. We had a bit of a strange way of communicating because of the 'language barrier' between us all.

When my brother Cameron was born, and mum was in hospital, she told dad to ask me to help locate things he couldn't find around the house. The strange thing was that I was only about 2½ years old at the time.

At playtime I was always very focused and had my ideas on how things were supposed to go no matter what, which was interesting for my parents. I wasn't very good at sharing, playing or giving things to my brother, which made him very frustrated at times. Being the firstborn I was used to having all the playthings being mine and not shared.

When he came along everything was different. He was the boy and I was the girl, but I was fascinated by his toys. He had much more interesting things like cars and soldiers to play with. I was a real tomboy who hated wearing skirts and dresses—I was made to wear them every Sabbath to church, which annoyed me so much.

One day we were both given presents. To my surprise I had been given a little red cowgirl's outfit with a skirt, while my brother got a black cowboy vest with a silver sheriff's star on it and black cowboy pants to go along with it. 'Whhaat! What! I want to have his outfit, mum! I don't want a skirt! Manny's [Cammy's] is better!' I bitterly complained to my mother.

'Now, now, Megs, there's no need to be like this—you'll look pretty in your red skirt and matching vest!' my mum soothingly said to me. I just glared at her until she took me up in her arms and gave me a big cuddle.

Well, after that just about every chance I got, I wore his black vest and black pants even though the pants were too small. I didn't want to be a girl and wear dresses. I wanted to be a boy instead, wearing jeans and anything denim. I didn't want to look like a prissy girl. I wanted to be me and only me!

We had some white tulle and a black jacket for dress-ups and my brother and I would take turns dressing up as the bride. Oh what fun times we had as kids! But there were frustrating times too.

As soon as I could speak I used my own language. Mum and dad called it Meganese, because they couldn't understand it. I was still quite fluent in it until I was about four years old when my parents started to call it rubbish talk and almost banned it.

Then came the weekly visit to a nice lady who spoke to me clearly and I was supposed to try to copy her. My parents told me that she was a speech therapist, and she would help me speak more clearly. She gave me a book filled with different sounds and a lot of colourful pictures and I was to practise these with my parents at home.

I never got into trouble for saying the wrong thing, but was always encouraged to say it right. In this book there were both prompts for my parents and me. At the time I had no idea why I was doing all this stuff but just accepted it as part of my life as an innocent child.

I had always felt I was somehow different to other children but I didn't know why. Sometimes I felt as if I were on some type of higher level and found it really hard to relate to other kids. I much preferred spending time and doing things with the grown-ups or adults around me. Perhaps it was because I got more stimulation and understanding from them, which I didn't when I was with other children.

The early years in my life were like a huge adventure for me and I had my own strong individual personality. I was so friendly and usually loved being around people; as a little tot I still had the occasional tantrum that I was of course disciplined for.

I generally had a happy nature. I had no idea then that I was going to fall through the cracks of life in the future. It wasn't until I started school that I began to lose my childhood innocence and not trust people and authority figures.

3

Primary School Daze—An Educational Fog

Sydney, 1982 onwards

Two of the bigger boys grabbed my hands. They took one each and I realised with horror that I was becoming a 10 year old human tug-of-war rope. It felt like I was being pulled apart as they spun me around several times.

This happened a couple of times at school with no teacher intervening. I hated it so much and I was so scared that they'd actually pull me in half and hurt me more. I was yelling out, 'Stop it please!' but no-one heard me. It just fell on deaf ears.

School! School was not a happy place for me at all. I found it very, very difficult indeed and my experiences at school had a great effect on me through to adulthood. I found everything about it difficult— different teachers, different schools, my problem communicating with others, and moving from interstate.

My earliest memories of the education system are when I started going to pre-school in a little Western Australian town called Geraldton. I remember that I was quite fussy about some things, which probably seemed quite strange to the other kids.

There is one day that still stands out vividly in my mind. I was only three or four years old. As I have mentioned, I hated wearing sleeveless dresses or shirts and I hated anyone wearing them. For some reason it made me feel so uncomfortable. On this particular day my mum dropped me off and when I entered the schoolyard I saw that one of the teachers had no sleeves in her dress, which freaked me out. I didn't want to be there so I turned around and walked out of the gate, and kept on walking, walking, walking, crossing streets on my way home. I was so determined to get home that I was like a little homing pigeon travelling along.

The temperature was about 43°C—quite normal there, but very hot for a little girl to be walking in. I must have walked about two or three kilometres along a reasonably deserted bush road when a lady who knew my parents stopped her car beside me. She must have wondered what this crazy little tot was doing here all by herself!

Hurriedly she bundled me into her car and drove me home immediately. When my parents saw me they got quite a fright because I could have been kidnapped. I remember I had a glass of milk and slept for hours because I was so exhausted after all that walking. I think I gave my parents their first few grey hairs that day!

I also remember feeling closer to some kindergarten teachers than others but I don't recall interacting with the other children very well. I am sure that over the years I have blocked out quite a few things because they were too painful for me at the time. Yet there are times when I can remember certain bits and pieces in clear detail. Thinking back I actually don't know how I survived school or the education system at all.

From Geraldton we moved to Esperance with my dad's work as a pastor. It was quite a small town and the church had a school there so the obvious thing was that I go to that school. So my first school had only about eight students with all grades combined in the one classroom and only one teacher teaching us all at the same time. I found him confusing. Maybe it was partly to do with the rules, which I didn't understand.

Every morning we would have devotions and prayer with all the other students. Another kid used to chew his fingernails all the time. I remember watching him doing it and being absolutely fascinated by it. So I started biting my nails too, just to be like him in some sense. One day we were all sitting down in a circle for the morning devotions and for some reason the teacher got annoyed with us for biting our fingernails. So afterwards he called me off into a separate room and gave me the cane, which was a reasonably small ruler. After the caning I was crying and really upset; why had this man hit me for no apparent reason? Afterwards we both knelt on the floor and he prayed with me for some reason that I can't remember. That was my first and unfortunately not the last experience of corporal punishment at school. When that happened it hurt me a lot and I began to not trust teachers as much.

From there I went to Kalgoorlie Public School, which had about 500 students in the school. The good part was that there were other teachers around all the time. The other kids didn't really understand me, which I found hard. I was new and could not communicate with them effectively. I remember one hit me over the head with a tennis racket, and some used rulers, but nothing hurt me for some reason. I was kind of proud of that. I was at least getting some kind of attention. We were only in Kalgoorlie for about nine months so it wasn't really enough time for me to bond properly with other people.

From Kalgoorlie we then had a huge move across country to the big city of Sydney and there I was, back in a very small school. The private school that my brother and I started attending had only about 15 students and one teacher for everyone. It was a vast change from my last school. We started at the very end of the school year in 1981. I was nine years old and was also put back a grade at the start of the new year, which I found really confusing. I realised later that this was only because of the different education systems of Western Australia and NSW.

The school was on quite a big bit of land although the actual schoolhouse was reasonably small. Next door there was a bigger school, separated by a high wire fence that you could see through clearly. So we could see what the other students from that school were doing during lunchtime and they could see us as well. It was around this time that I started getting teased and hassled at school again. But it was heaps worse than it was before!

I don't know how it happened but over the next two years nearly the whole school ganged up on me, especially the boys. They started calling me names, which I hated. They kept on at me and wouldn't stop it even for a second. I had no support from the teacher at all and I used to lose my temper, and start running around shouting and hooting, trying to make the other kids stop it. The kids from the school next door used to see this as well on nearly a daily basis.

They too would flock around the fence and watch what was happening. A few of them used to join in with the kids from my school, cheering. I didn't understand this at the time but all my running around was only making it worse for myself. But what was I supposed to do when no-one else was standing up for me including my teacher and my brother? I remember that I was so angry with everything going on that I hit my brother a few times at school one day with something, which I think I did get into trouble for. Poor little guy; he didn't understand what was going on either.

This was when I was 'IT'—becoming the tug-of-war rope itself.

What was worse, I never told my parents what was happening until many years later when I started exhibiting quite strange and disturbed behaviour that worried my family a lot.

In this school there was also a 15-year-old Down syndrome boy. I didn't like him that much at all because at lunchtime he used to chase me all over the yard trying to catch me for some reason that I didn't understand. This really, really scared me a lot and yet our teacher seemed to do nothing about it. Quite often she had lunch in her office, which was inside the building. Or she could have been having her lunch in the schoolhouse. I don't remember her supervising us children much during those times. After lunch she would read us a book and we would all sit on the floor listening to her.

Another time I was playing with a bug-catcher trying to catch bees or butterflies in the schoolyard and for some reason it annoyed my teacher. I didn't know why. She took it off me, dragged me into her office and gave me the cane, which was a feather duster or ruler. This really confused me as I didn't understand why I got the cane just for playing as all kids do. It seemed to be just another one of the strange things with this school.

During this time I was severely depressed and deeply homesick for everyone over in Western Australia. At night I used to have trouble staying asleep so in the middle of the night or early in the morning I would turn on my bed light and read different books for hours on end. For some reason I'd make little rips in some of the pages of my books.

Also on the way to and from school I started collecting leaves, stones, sticks, branches or whatever else took my fancy and putting them into plastic bags that I had with me. I remember walking along the road and seeing things with a colour, shape or texture I liked, such as a yellowy type of leaf or a small stick with an interesting mark on it or a small smooth stone. I would stuff these into my school case, then empty it out under my bed when I got home. Imagine how surprised my mother was when she went to clean my bedroom!

I was fascinated by words, names, and number plates among other things at that time, and on the way to and from school I would draw faces and islands. I used to do a lot of humming as well—Christian songs or classical music over and over, which I quite liked. A few other people around me on the buses used to get quite annoyed about it and tell me off. When that happened I used to go really quiet and wanted to cry because I felt so bad. The humming for me was a way to let things out and amuse myself on the bus rides, but other people found my behaviour quite strange.

I also liked talking to a few older people who used the bus quite regularly. Sometimes in Warriewood several Italian people would get on the bus in the afternoons. I used to sit down where they were and talk to one or two of the middle-aged women. I enjoyed myself because they seemed to like me and were nice to me. I'd look forward to the days when they were on the bus. A few Asian students also got on at Narrabeen. Once, one or two of the girls wrote down my name in Korean.

A couple of the other kids from school didn't understand why I talked to the older people, especially George, who was always really cheeky and smart all the time. He used to call some of the girls 'Fatty Boomsticks' and 'Skinny Bangsticks' and other names. He was one of the guys at school who used to tease me mercilessly.

In the middle of winter we had to train for the long-distance running and other events for the school sports carnival. I had an extremely bad cold that made me feel really sick, but it didn't matter to my teacher. She would make all of us run around the school fence line and if we stopped running and started walking for whatever reason we got into trouble. It was not very comfortable running in very slippery school shoes up a slippery slope around a very big yard for lap upon lap upon lap … maybe 10 laps or more. I can't remember.

The Down syndrome boy was behind me some of the times, running, and I used to try to run or jog fast so he couldn't catch me because I was so scared that he was going to do something bad to me. I used to go home from school sicker than when I left. Funny, but I can't remember if I told my parents that. I'm not sure whether I used deodorant either so I must have been a bit on the nose at times without realising it. I wasn't in a good way at all.

I was at this school for just over three years. I remember having crushes or liking one or two of the boys there and once they found this out, the teasing got heaps worse. I think I cried but I'm not too sure. I just felt really left out.

I would try to join in by playing soccer or cricket with the other kids. When the soccer ball slammed into my shins I didn't mind, because I felt like part of something. It was the same with cricket when I used to hit the tennis ball really long distances. I was quite strong and very tall for my age so I found that heaps of fun. Brandings was a game I hated and avoided because the other kids used it as a way to pick on me.

Once Rebecca, who was an older girl at the school, looked over the toilet stall when I was going to the toilet. She was saying some not very nice things and it really freaked me out about using the toilets there. Even today I still hate public toilets because of this incident.

I felt so alone during this time, with all this stuff going on. But what kept me going was looking at the birds in the sky and nature all around. I remember as we walked to the bus stop we'd get over the crest of the hill and see Warriewood valley. There were small farms and bush and I used to love looking at the afternoon sun shining on everything. I found it really peaceful amid all the turmoil that was going on in my life.

At the beginning of 1984 things changed a bit with a brand new teacher called Mrs Brighteyes. I thought she was a really nice teacher and I liked her a lot ... until I heard her singing voice! My reaction was over the top to say the least. I would hunch down and try to cover my ears. To me the sound of her singing was like hearing someone scratch their fingernails down a blackboard. I absolutely hated it. The poor teacher must have thought I was mad with this extreme reaction.

My parents were extremely worried about my behaviour and took me to see a specialist in ADD and minimal brain dysfunction, which I had been diagnosed with when I was seven. He diagnosed ADD and then prescribed Ritalin tablets to help me.

Mrs Brighteyes asked me to stand up in front of the whole school as she explained my condition. Afterwards she encouraged the other kids to ask questions about what I had. I felt really awkward and embarrassed about the whole situation.

At least with Mrs Brighteyes things were a bit better at school. I liked listening to her read books aloud and the other creative types of activities she planned for us. I remember once for biblical studies we were to write our version of a parable that Jesus told, then read it out in class the week after. I was so excited about this that I decided to make mine really interesting.

I had been reading about a group of Hell's Angels bikies in a magazine in the waiting room of one of the several doctors my parents had been taking me to at this time. So what I did was make up a story of a gang of bikers in the sand dunes and a lady who came walking along. She was attacked and then gang-raped by all the bikers, then just left there. When she tried to get help from a couple of other people they said, 'No!' Yet there was a good biker in the group who saw what happened, rescued her and took her to safety. So he was the modern day Good Samaritan.

I thought that it was a good story but when it came time to handing it in to the teacher, I absolutely refused. There was a tug of war over my book before she eventually got it from me. She must have read it to herself because after that she called my parents in for a talk. I remember I was outside when they were talking. It seemed to go on for a long time.

Primary school had been full of horrors and misunderstandings, but I had no idea that high school could be worse.

4

High School Hiccups

[Megan] has started mutilating herself again. All these activities are both disturbing to the rest of the class and time-consuming for the staff involved and cannot be allowed to continue. Hence she has been placed on a one-day suspension ...
— letter from my high school principal just after my 15th birthday

By the time I reached high school, a private Christian school for all levels, I was in a bad way socially because of many things that had happened already in my life and which I will deal with later. I found it nearly impossible to relate to any of the other kids around me, which was really hard. The teachers, as the excerpt of the letter from the principal above shows so clearly, had no idea how to handle me either, with all my myriad problems. It would be over 10 years—turbulent years for me and my family—before I had the final diagnosis and knew what was causing me so much distress.

I didn't trust anyone at all and found myself getting into fights with some of the boys in Years 6 and 7. I felt so alone and was so angry with everything that was going on. I found myself with a severe hair-pulling habit that left me with so many bald patches that I had to wear a beret out of school hours because I was so embarrassed. My fingernails were also quite often bitten down so much that I'd pull out the quicks and had sticking plasters all over my fingers sometimes.

I got into lots of trouble with the teachers; getting demerit points, lunchtime and afternoon detentions, and in-school suspensions. The teachers had no real idea what was going on with me. I had no idea what was going on with me either! I was a little enigma to everyone around me, including myself.

By the time I was about 14 years old I was feeling suicidal and I'd quite often think about killing myself in some way, shape or form. I'd also started self-destructive activities like self-mutilating by cutting myself repeatedly with one of mum's sharp kitchen knives, and bashing myself nearly senseless with rulers.

This is a poem that I wrote when I was in high school, which really describes how I felt.

One Sad Lonely Person

One sad, lonely person walking down the cobblestones of life.
Not content, too afraid of what's going to become of him.
Feeling sad, feeling lonely
Sitting on the chair of judgement.
A ringing of a bell, the ping of rain.
Too sad to go anywhere.
Like a bird in a cage
Trying to free himself from the cage of life—
Flying freely with no worries, no cares.
A life of happiness extends its hands to
The tired and weary traveller of life
Who was caged up like a bird
And is now as happy as a bird.

© Megan Hammond, 1986

When I was in Year 10 the school put out an annual magazine and the students were encouraged to submit things. I wrote four poems and put them in and to my surprise they were published, which was really big for me because part of me was finally beginning to be noticed. Although the poems didn't rhyme or anything, it still meant a lot to have them read. This poem expresses how alone I felt at school a lot of the time.

Alone

Alone in a big open room I sit
Watching everyone about me
Their faces cold and harsh
Their bodies are statues.
Alone through the yard I walk
Seeing people talking everywhere
Their faces warm and friendly one moment
But uninviting and cold the next.
Alone through the darkness of life
I see ghostly white shadows ignoring me
They see me then they turn away,
And their faces haunt me.
Alone I am forced to be
With no friends in the world
Their images ugly and contorted
Haunt me like ghosts in the night.

©Megan Hammond, 1989

I had not read this poem for many years and it brought back to me how hard I did find school. Year 10 was the final year of school for me—I left in 1989. I was always one of the oldest in my classes at school because of my developmental difficulties. Without the capacity to communicate with teachers or other students effectively I was way behind, and it was decided it would be best for all if I left. I could never have coped with the stress or workload of Years 11 and 12.

The final year of high school was especially turbulent for me. I was a rebel without a cause in a Christian school. All the other girls were goody-two-shoes types; Christian girls who stuck together in cliques. Sometimes I did hang around with one or two other girls, but not often. I was bullied by the boys in my class on different levels. I found it hard, but kept going.

Vanessa was one of the girls I used to hang around with from time to time. Vanessa had a blonde bobbed hairstyle. She was really intelligent and quite a good friend. She probably found it hard to understand what was going on with me at the time but we had a few fun times and really good talks. One day I had a packet of cigarettes in my bag.

This day she came up to me in a real hurry saying, 'I've heard the teachers are going to do a big check for contraband! You better do something with the cigarettes!'

My stunned reply was, 'What! I don't believe it! Are you sure?'

'Yes, of course!' came her reply.

So I quickly got my cigarettes and hurriedly took them to the toilets to try to dispose of the evidence. She stood out the front standing guard. I locked myself in the cubicle and tried to flush the cigarettes down the toilet without much success. The bloody things kept on popping up and floating after being flushed. In the toilet bowl all you could see were bits and pieces of broken cigarettes, whole cigarettes and tobacco mixed in with a bit of toilet paper that I used to try to get it down better. The fear of being caught rushed through me because I didn't want to be suspended yet again, or worse, expelled!

Eventually all the evidence had flushed away, including the cigarette packet. I hope it didn't block the drains up. I walked outside to Vanessa and told her, 'Hey! I've got rid of all the cigarettes in the toilet!'

She sighed, turned towards me and said something like, 'Glad to hear that! Make sure you don't bring cigarettes to school again because they're bad for you!'

'Yes, Vanessa, okay,' was my embarrassed reply.

Looking back on it I have to have a bit of a smile about how wild I actually was.

~

The year 1988 was a heartbreaker of a year for our whole family in more ways than one. Every aspect of my life was in a state of confusion. The family's world had been tipped upside down too. In January we went on a family holiday back to Western Australia for the first time since we left there in November 1981. It meant a lot to see so many friends and family, whom we hadn't seen in years.

One day in February both my parents came to the school at the end of the day to get my brother and me. As soon as I saw mum I felt worried because she looked really teary. 'Kids!' they said, 'we've just found out that Nana is dead!' Their words trailed off into nothingness as my mind went into shock. None of us could believe it because we'd only seen her, my mother's mum, a few weeks before and she had seemed fine.

In the space of that year from February 1988 to February 1989, five family members or friends died—including Keleb, the family dog. I kept on getting into trouble at school with demerit points, detentions and so on. At home I was having arguments with my parents and was permanently attached to the record player, listening to my records with headphones on. And I was self-harming, which wasn't good. I became really depressed.

I was just not a happy Vegemite! At the time I was seeing a counsellor at Queenscliff Health Centre with my family to try to work things out. My poor parents and I had no idea why I was so different and causing so much anxiety for everyone around me.

Twice I ran away from home. Once I walked out of school and ended up in a suburb a couple of kilometres away.

It was straight after this that my counsellor suggested that I join a program at Dalwood Children's Home to try to sort things out. My parents and I were at desperation point and would've done anything to make our family work better, so plans were made immediately for me to go to the unit at Dalwood in Seaforth. I would stay there during the week and come home to my parents on the weekends. I found freedom at Dalwood that I'd never felt at home! No holds barred. We got more pocket money to spend on things. We didn't have to worry about parents. Oh you could do so many more things at Dalwood than you ever did at home!

'Dalwood—The Place To Be!' would have been the slogan for an advertising poster in my mind.

I met Lisa at Dalwood, and Annabel and Andrew were also there. Those kids were really interesting and the place felt better than home because the rules were less strict there.

After a while Lisa was teaching me how to smoke cigarettes properly by actually inhaling the smoke. She used to call my way of smoking 'bum puffs' because I never used to inhale. I held the smoke inside my mouth. I used to get really bad headaches and feel very dizzy—head spins. Lisa was this really cool goth chick with dusty blonde, shortish, messy hair, who wore dark eyeliner all the time.

She also wrote poetry and her handwriting looked really gothic and funny. We liked the same music and we always used to talk late into the night. I found myself being drawn to her in a mysterious elusive way. I wanted to be close to her and I remember once we were on her bed listening to music. We fell asleep and gave each other a hug and held hands. That time when I was beside her I felt so comfortable and really safe. It was like we were linked almost, and were kindred spirits.

I found myself drawn deeper to her somehow and I often wondered if she felt the same way. I never had the guts to ask her if she did or act on my feelings in case I got rejected. Anyway, she seemed pretty keen on guys. She was about a year younger than me but there was something about her. There were many times my lips were so drawn to hers yet I respected her and I was too shy, and also young, like her.

I was 15 years old when we met at Dalwood. She was troubled like me but I still was really attracted to her. I was having all these feelings that were new and strange to me.

Sometimes we were taken on different activities at night with some of the counsellors, including going for a swim at Manly in the middle of winter. It was so cold, but loads of fun. Other times we went to a cafe in Balgowlah that served different coffees.

'Now what type of coffee would everyone like?' asked the waitress standing at the table before us. Looking through the interesting list of all these different coffees I'd never tasted before was mesmerising. In the end I chose Vienna coffee and the others ordered theirs. We all sat around the table with the Dalwood staff that were on duty that night. I was feeling really excited because I hadn't tried this coffee before—we didn't drink it very much at home as a family.

Our coffees came out and I saw that mine had a bit of froth on top of it. It tasted really bitter and awful so I put a bit more sugar in it. It was my first taste of coffee—too strong for me! I remember coming away with a bad but interesting taste in my mouth.

Talking about bad tastes in my mouth I remember having a huge argument with my counsellor one day at Dalwood. 'Why have you locked yourself in your room?' Jane's exasperated voice came through the door.

I was sitting hunched up with my back wedged against it thinking, 'I don't want to speak to my counsellor! I want to be left alone!' After more talking I did eventually open up my door and Jane was waiting for me.

As soon as I walked out I could see that she wasn't too impressed with what I had done. I was so embarrassed that I was looking down at the floor as she was talking to me. Her eyes were burning a hole into my head and I felt that I was only 10 centimetres tall. Being the typical teenager I tried to put on a tough front but I was shaking in my boots because I hated discipline and being told off. My communication style back then was more immature than most kids my age and in high school it was causing me a whole lot more problems, which I hated.

During the school holidays, just after my 16th birthday, a group of us was taken to Forster-Tuncurry for a camp with a couple of counsellors from Dalwood. It was at this time that some things would happen in my life that would change me forever.

We were away for about a week and a half. One night we met two guys who were staying at the same caravan park we were. They had been drinking quite a bit and Lisa started talking to them. I was there just trying to also take part in the conversation. Still talking, we walked to the beach, then Lisa started kissing this guy that she was with; I saw her on the sand with him. Then Nick, the guy I was with, started kissing me. Things started getting heated between both couples. Nick put his towel on the beach and we lay down together, and I ended up losing my virginity to him. I don't think he got it all the way in and nothing much happened because it was way too painful for me.

The next day I remember walking up the beach and sitting down in great pain, feeling really confused about things. We agreed not to tell the counsellors or workers what had happened and to try to forget about it. When we were leaving to go back to Sydney, we said goodbye to the guys, but it all stayed with me. I did it to get close to Lisa as much as anything, because I wanted her to accept me and like me more.

Remember, this was the 1980s. In the media there was a lot of hype about the Grim Reaper and people getting AIDS through unsafe sex as well as other things. I was worried that I could've got AIDS because I wasn't protected. About a month later I asked my mum something like, 'Can you still get it even if the guy didn't come or ejaculate inside you?'

She said, 'Yes. Why? Have you done something?'

Then it all came out and I was sitting down in the lounge room with my parents talking about it. The memory of the whole conversation is blurred but they were saying things like, 'You don't want to be like a dog and have sex with just anyone that comes past. You can't be promiscuous and sleep around.' I felt they were calling me a slut. 'You're supposed to wait until you are married,' they said.

Dad said that in three months he would take me to a clinic in Surry Hills for an HIV or AIDS test. I was absolutely petrified, out of my mind because I was so scared that I might have actually caught it from that 'Nick off!' guy as mum called him.

It was at this time that I decided not to ever talk to my parents about my sex life again because it hurt so much. These were the longest three months of my life ever. I had the test done and waited a week for the results. They came back negative and I was so relieved. I was determined not to have unsafe sex ever again!

~

Some of the boys at school were cruel and unforgiving, which was really hard to deal with. They harassed me with crude suggestions, which eventually led to more.

A few guys gave me a really hard time. I was too young to realise what was really going on at the time. They would pick on me all the time saying really belittling things, shoving or punching me sometimes. Nothing seemed to make them happy. One of them used to say, 'You're frigid aren't you! C'mon!?' Then he'd quite often try to touch me. This would happen quite a lot.

The boys saw me as different from the other girls so they picked on me severely. Seeing my weakness and social vulnerability they attacked mercilessly, like a pack of wolves devouring my soul alive.

I used to get into fights with the boys at school because they hassled me so much. One time a boy punched me in the stomach. I was winded and doubled over in so much pain but got no sympathy from the other boys. I hated it.

Wolfie was one of the main offenders. When I was 16, he somehow found out that I wasn't a virgin any more and his jeering got even worse. In about February or March of that year we had ice-skating for sport in a nearby suburb. He kept on at me, saying, 'Why don't you prove it? Why don't you prove you're not frigid?'

His grandparents lived in the area and we organised to meet up after sport time. A week later we ended up hiding near a tree and I did some sexual stuff to him. I couldn't stand it and I was afraid that we were going to get caught but he kept pushing me on. I was hating it, but he seemed to enjoy it. I caught the bus feeling disgusted with myself and crept home.

Another week we went to his grandparents' house where more things happened with no disturbances. He wanted to have sex with me and I replied, 'Not without a condom, I don't want to get pregnant!'

'Okay, that's cool! I don't think I've got anything but I'll try to find something!'

He then rummaged about the house and found a small plastic bag that he put on himself. I was feeling dead scared and didn't want to go along with it but I found myself going through the actions. He tried to do stuff that wasn't working, put soap or something on the bag which stung me, and he managed to do it much to my disgust.

We got dressed, left the house and went our own ways back home. I remember sitting on the bus on the way home feeling like a used, sad and sore rag doll. My stomach was nauseous and I hated what had just happened between us. I thought I was acting like a dog or animal as my parents implied when I first lost my virginity! Or that I was being un-Christian and having sex before marriage.

My train of thought was: What on earth have I done? I'm so stupid! I can never tell my mum and dad about what happened because they'll kill me. From what happened the last time I can't share this with them!

Until I had written this book my parents didn't know that ever happened and it is something that I try not to think about too often. The consequences of what happened flooded through my school life nearly drowning me in it.

For the rest of that year it was hell on Earth. Wolfie basically ignored me at school and we never spoke about what had happened between us. I think he called me a 'slut' or a 'dog' a few times. For no apparent reason the teasing from him and his mates got worse, and I felt so low. He probably bragged about it to his mates without me knowing … I have no idea. I saw one of the few people I felt I could trust, the school counsellor, a few times about losing my virginity and a few other issues, but never told her about what happened with Wolfie and me.

I felt really betrayed and hurt because I was hoping the situation would improve, but it never did. I felt like such an outcast because all the other girls still had their virginity and they were being good Christian girls and I was the totally stupid one who fell. I also remember thinking that I never wanted anything like this to happen to me again!

The end of Year 10, the end of school for me, was nearing and I was greatly looking forward to it. It meant that I no longer was going to be around those bullies who were always so cruel to me.

I experienced many different and new emotions about leaving the Christian school I had been attending. I was sick to death of the rules and regulations, and wanted to be free at last. On one of the last weekends before school finished I figured I'd get my ears pierced for a second time. This was against the school's very strict rules about jewellery, but after all, what could 'they'—the teachers—do so close to the end? I found out.

What happened next surprised both my parents and me completely. The principal and staff decided to put me on a four-day in-school suspension. I had to sit in the library and do my normal class work. The reason was that I had already skipped between three and five afternoon after-school detentions by sneaking up to the school buses and slipping through the net of schoolteachers. I was the fish who kept getting away and they were determined to catch me no matter what!

My 'pond' was a study room in the library with a big clear window to the librarian's office up the front. The librarian was the sort of person who could see all and hear all. She could hear a pin drop in the study room next door. Her tall figure was a bit plump and quite intimidating to a teenager like me.

When my parents heard about my suspension they had a huge discussion with some of the staff and then the principal gave me a stern talking to. After a day or so I was let off from doing the rest of it, luckily. I could've spent my last days in the study room away from all my friends and the people that I wasn't going to see for much longer.

During the last few days the whole school turned out for the giving-out of our Year 10 certificates and to say farewell to those who were leaving that year. After all the formalities we signed each other's shirts and school yearbooks. Then came the class formal that night; the last time we would be united as a class. There was an after-party at someone's house and there was a bit of underage drinking but who cared anyway?

'School's out.' The words from this Alice Cooper song came to mind. School IS out forever ... It is finished! Literally forever!

A new, different and scary world awaited me—the world of work, bosses, pay packets, budgets and fellow employees. My journey through the education system had been hard, but maybe this new world of work would be understanding, even welcoming, to this dispirited teenager. It was like I had an unknown force or mysterious weakness following me all the time. It wasn't until years later that I found out it was called Asperger's syndrome.

There was the possibility of a job for me through mum's work at the Spastic Centre. The job going was as an electronics assembler or process worker on the line with non-cerebral palsy people. It seemed pretty interesting so I went for it because it meant money. Mum recommended me to the manager of that department. Walking into the room of my first job interview was scary. Memories of career training classes at school went through my head.

'Good morning! You must be Megan Hammond ... Sally's daughter?' This tall figure came out from behind his desk with his hand extended welcomingly.

'Yes! Hello, I'm Megan. Nice to meet you,' I nervously said as I shook his hand. Wow, he's like a giant, this guy! I can't believe it! I thought to myself, in awe of his size.

We sat down and began the interview that changed the next few years of my life ...

5

Juggling Jobs

K ching! Crack! went the board as it came onto my console. Diodes, resistors, ICs and LEDs, among other components, were spaced everywhere throughout the board. The diagram that was meant to help me was like a puzzle itself. If you put it upside down or the other way around you'd be in a big mess. Then I had to pick up the next board and start again. The process work went on and on and ...

I found out really quickly why it was called process work. The electronics assembly line was one of my most boring jobs.

I've had many types of work in my life. My first part-time job was when I was in primary school where I helped mum with kitchen work in the vegetarian pie factory she had. My brother and I also helped out in one of her health food shops, which was interesting. During the school holidays at high school I worked as a volunteer carer for the Spastic Centre.

On the daily outings I would help push people's wheelchairs, talking and spending time with them and feeding them too. I did find being with them fun in a way. At that time I was also a part-time kitchen hand with mum when she did cooking lessons once a week at Sydney Adventist Hospital, which I also liked doing. My work was probably a bit slower than most people's. Also, during Year 10, I had done a couple of weeks' work experience at a local hairdressing salon. I was slow and didn't really know how to show initiative.

Working at the Spastic Centre was hugely different from school but in a good way, because I was getting paid. It gave me a chance to start spending money and to save for a family trip overseas to America and Europe in September of that year, 1990. In April of that year the centre started retrenching many workers there, including me, because they were eventually closing that section down.

Now I was out of work, looking for new work and happened to find a job a bit later that month just up the road from the Spastic Centre.

This job was quite different because not only did I have to put the electronic components in, I had to solder all the backs of them on the circuit board. It took ages to hand solder each and every little joint. Sometimes when I got bored I used to get all the small metal spikes or whatever and join them up with solder so that it looked like a metal spider web—I tried to be careful not to get caught doing that. I would get the clippers, then clip the spikes really short as we were supposed to do, check the back and front, then put it on the finished tray.

While I had been working at the Spastic Centre, I noticed I had difficulty relating to people and understanding different things, but I had no idea how to deal with that. Now at my new job I was noticing that:

- I had trouble asking questions and communicating with my superiors if I had any trouble with the work I was doing.
- I had trouble listening to, taking and understanding verbal instructions because it was easier for me if they were written down. Having a diagram of the particular circuit board we were working on at the time showing where all the components went was easier.
- I found the job very, very repetitive and thus very boring for me, so I looked for other ways of amusing myself—hence the additional soldering.
- I found it very tiring sitting there all day doing work without moving

around much except during the breaks and at lunchtimes.

- I had no real idea about the speed I should be working at. I was going at my own pace and trying my best to complete the boards properly, which happened to be slower than everyone around me.
- I didn't understand or comprehend the concept of getting the different orders done in the specific time frame or how important it was.
- I was like a fish out of water in a lot of different ways.

In August, not long before the overseas trip, I was retrenched because the company was having financial troubles. It wasn't until I got back from the holiday some time in October that I discovered the company had finally closed down. For the next five to 10 years electronics companies with process work were closing down all over Australia for various reasons. One of the main reasons was because it was much cheaper to get the work done in Asia. So in fact I was part of a dying industry and that explains the loss of my jobs and other people's jobs in the process.

After the holiday, and unemployed for the second time that year, I soon joined up with the CES and Social Security to try and find work. The reality was, I had no real job skills for other types of work. I hated this. It wasn't until halfway through 1991 that Alex, my first serious boyfriend, found us part-time evening jobs, only a few nights a week, because a guy he knew needed help at his pasta restaurant. I became the pasta cook and Alex helped Victor, his mate, with waiting tables out the front.

Being the pasta cook was quite easy because there was basically one type of pasta, which was fresh spaghetti, with about seven or eight ready-made sauces to put on top of it. We had to put garlic spread on the bread and heat them up as needed. During the busy times on Friday and Saturday nights we'd get about 70 to 100 customers, or even more, on each of those nights. By the end of the night we helped clean and shut down the shop and we would be so tired it wasn't funny. We both found the work hard yet quite satisfying.

We'd quite often ride our pushbikes back to my parents' house; it was so cold during the winter nights, especially at that hour. Alex would then ride back to his parents' house after that.

I managed to save up for a brand new mountain bike, which I really needed for transport. The day Alex and I went to get it I was so proud and happy with myself. We both worked with Victor until about November when the restaurant eventually closed down, which was sad.

One day Alex said to me, 'I know what we can do, Megan! We can be volunteer counsellors for a week at a blind camp at Crosslands. What do you think?'

My reply was, 'Wow, Alex! I've never really thought about that. Is it going to be hard to do?'

'No of course not!' was Alex's answer to that. 'It's going to be quite easy guiding blind people around doing different things! Besides, I think we get a couple of days of training.'

So that sealed it. We both sent our forms in and were accepted as volunteers. That week was really interesting, but hard in a few ways for me. I hadn't been back to Crosslands since something bad had happened to me there in 1985, so memories were coming back to haunt me. I was not used to helping someone else on such a close and intimate level for a whole week either, so at the end of the week I just sat down and cried for about an hour or so, letting it all out. I could see the parallels. Here I was helping a young blind woman, while I was equally blind to relating to people properly. During this time I did see a very different side of life, which meant something to me.

Then in May 1992 a friend of Alex's family gave me a casual cleaning job at the company he was working for. It turned out to be once a week at a huge clothing warehouse and sorting place, run through Wesley Central Mission. My instructions were to clean, mop all the toilets and the little kitchen area, and vacuum everywhere on the floor where the clothing was. It was a monumental task that was put before me and I don't think I was given a real time frame. I took it literally, vacuuming all around the workstations and moving everything back and forth to get everything clean. By the end of the day I was exhausted, but I knew I tried my best. It wasn't until two months later when I left to do the hospitality course at the Human Resources Centre run though the CES that I realised I had been a lot more thorough than the other cleaners had been.

Over the next year I did two back-to-back, six-month courses to try to get more skills. The first one was a very basic hospitality course, then in 1993 I did an ATY Understanding Children course. I didn't get a certificate for it because I failed a couple of subjects. Actually it was because I failed to hand in a few assignments that were part of the assessment. Come to think of it I never managed to complete any assignments at school either!

Coming out of those courses with a bit more experience, I soon found a job in July 1993 at a childcare centre where I worked as an assistant for a year. Not long before Christmas I was bending and twisting to get something from a bottom cupboard. Something went crack in my knee and I ended up hurting it really badly. I was taken to the doctor and was informed that I had to take a break from work until the knee healed more.

I ended up on crutches for a few weeks, which I found really annoying. For a couple of months I wore a bandage around my knee but unfortunately it was never the same again. It actually still gives me quite a bit of pain so I have to be careful what I do with it. After the school and Christmas holidays I went back to work with a bandaged leg and met the new owners of the centre. I really did love the work and the little kids there but it was quite stressful as it was a long day-care centre. As always I had the same little problems of not showing enough initiative. I was so upset when, later on that year, in June 1994, I had to leave. I loved everything about the place, but nothing could be done.

About a month after leaving there I found a job again as an electronics assembler at Cochlear, well known for developing hearing aid implants. This was a much bigger place than I was used to and a lot finer detail was required in the work. It was meant to be contract work. I was on trial for three months, with the view to longer employment. I felt like a fish out of water again starting there, and I was also having a lot of changes and problems in my personal life. I found it so hard to adjust to all the new people around me. Then my parents left for a six-week trip to America, which really shook me up. Only later would I understand why change of any sort had always been so hard for me to tolerate.

Again at work the same problems with communication and understanding arose, which stressed me out because I felt so alone that I couldn't share it with anyone. I'd also developed a mad crush on another woman who worked in another area of the building, which made me even more confused about my sexuality.

In late 1994, not long after my parents got back from their trip, I was feeling very low and isolated. The pressure got too much for me to bear and I left a note on two friends' desks and attempted suicide in a local park through an overdose of sleeping tablets and muscle relaxants. This was my second attempt, but fortunately again people helped me. Just in time my friends had read the notes and, guessing where I would be, had rushed after me.

I ended up in hospital, returning to work a couple of days later. During one lunch hour I was driving up the road to get a pink slip for my car when another car slammed into the back of me. I was waiting to turn right when I heard a dreadful screech of brakes and felt a huge thump in the car. The other driver was a P-plate driver doing about 70kmh. I bumped my head in the crash and sat there stunned, bent and twisted, still sitting in the car. On the opposite corner was a cafe, and a few diners who saw the whole thing came out to help. I was dazed, in shock, and someone called my boss, who came to get me.

I had a very bad case of whiplash and was instantly off work under workers' compensation. Dosed up with painkillers and wearing a neck brace constantly for a couple of months, life for me at that stage seemed to be getting worse and more dramatic. I had great trouble trying to understand what was happening to me.

Feeling like I was letting the company down with my injury I was determined somehow to get back to work before Christmas. My old car was a total write-off but luckily I got money back from the insurance company, which was what I needed. With the help of my dearest dad I got my second car, another second-hand car, but I didn't mind that.

After that I did the most stupid thing just so I could go back to work with all my friends before Christmas. When I went to visit the doctor I lied and told him that I was a lot better when I actually wasn't at all. I was still in a huge amount of pain but didn't want to let the company down a couple of weeks before Christmas. So it was organised that I should go back to work, and I expected that everything was going to be the same again.

On the first day back at work I was welcomed warmly by my friends and I started doing my usual duties. Sometime in the morning I was called to the lady who ran the personnel office. I came in, sat down quietly, then heard the familiar words, 'Megan, there is something that we have to tell you ...'

She followed this by saying that they had to let me go for various reasons. It felt like a bomb had exploded in the room and I was in the centre of it. I don't remember much after that because I was in huge shock, but somehow I managed to leave the building and get to my car. Without thinking, I got behind the wheel and began driving. I didn't care where. I just wanted to get away. I had forgotten that my parents would be beside themselves with worry, especially when they discovered where I had been. But more of that later.

~

During the first few months of 1995 I moved out of home for the first time in my life—to Petersham with some people I knew. I couldn't find any work there but I did sign up for a part-time hospitality course that I never finished because my life turned upside down yet again.

It was July by the time I'd started another electronics assembling job in Artarmon. I found it hard to adjust to all the different people as well as the increased workload and I wasn't supported back at home with my new partner. At this time the relationship started getting more abusively violent in every way so my mind wasn't really on the job. Memories of hassles I'd had with other jobs were also coming back and this really worried me a lot. My partner also started causing problems by making prank phone calls to my workplace, which I was most uncomfortable with.

A few months later I was called into the office and retrenched. It was really distressing to be jobless once again and looking for work. I came back home where my partner and a friend were sitting around absolutely stoned. They started hurling abuse at me. I remember feeling so alone, hurt and confused, and I wished I was dead, gone, or somewhere else. I wanted to escape this thing called my life and I didn't know how it had become so bad so quickly.

~

The next month I became an internal sales clerk doing a traineeship at a medical equipment company. Being there was a huge new experience because not only did I have to deal with co-workers, learn everything in their 200-page medical catalogue, take orders and deal with phone customers putting in orders; every few weeks to a month there would be a staff assessment and also the completion of an evaluation form. After the form was filled in there was generally a short meeting and talk with management on how to improve. It was at that time I discovered that my people skills were below average. I thought this was probably because I was more used to dealing with printed circuit boards that didn't talk back to me, but it was, of course, my Asperger's.

Recently I found a supervisor's assessment report from the company and it reveals a lot. Here's a bit of it ...

Knowledge of duties described in job description: Below average

Competency at performing duties: Below average

Attention to detail: Below average

Telephone skills (where appropriate): Unsatisfactory

Performing to capacity: Average
Positive attitude: Average
Attendance and punctuality record: Above average

It was like a school report card—the first written feedback I'd had in six years. It was good to have because at least I now had everything down in writing and could understand what they were saying to me about my work. I liked receiving feedback like that and also supporting strategies on how to improve. At the time that wasn't enough. Over those months my personal life had become a living hell, which compounded the problems that I had at work.

After my partner wrote off my car, we broke up and I moved back home. I was now without transport and a long way from my work but that hardly mattered as a few days later I was called into the office and they told me that they had to let me go. I was in total shock because I had lost absolutely everything in the space of a few weeks. I was totally devastated to say the very least! The rest of 1995 was a total write off, like my car.

Finally, in November, I found a printed circuit board inspector job, which in a sense saved me. All the issues of meeting new people, starting a new job, finding public transport there, getting into a different schedule, all the usual things, came up again. My life was such a mess. I was sinking instead of swimming, grieving the loss of the relationship, my sleeping patterns were way out of whack, and I was smoking a pack of cigarettes a day. Out of work hours I was drinking heavily and to top it all a sleazy guy at work was trying to take advantage of me because I was so vulnerable.

I was a shell of my former self and quite underweight. My soul seemed to have escaped my body to get away from the constant violence and abuse. My mind was also trying to lose itself through alcohol, which I was using as a means of escape and to forget everything that had ever happened to me. At the end of that year, through staff general meetings, it was made clear to everyone that the company was having financial problems even though we were all working hard. Sometime in January 1997 the familiar call from the office was made. Once again I was told that they had to let me go!

Again, I was so upset about this bad cycle I was in of employers rejecting me all the time. I was so sure something was wrong with me and I had no hell of an idea what! It was only later that I found out that this company, yes another electronics company, had closed its doors. I had come to the end of my tether and completely given up on jobs and work. I'd always tried my best and put my soul into working and being a good worker, but the employers never seemed to understand or appreciate me at all. That was the turning point for me because all my trust in them was gone. Everything had got too much for me. They had completely beaten me and I was broken!

Since that time I have never had a paid full-time job again.

These experiences really scarred me to the core. Over the next few years I helped mum out sometimes with office work when I felt okay to do it. In 2000 I did work experience, organised through the CRS, for about two months at a video store. During those couple of months I felt so alive and needed. It was a good boost to my self-esteem being around positive people who were helping me.

The year after that, in 2001, I started doing voluntary work in Manly one or two days a week at the Community Aid Abroad shop, before my personal problems started to get in the way again. I was seeing someone who turned out to be not good for me, then we broke up. I did voluntary work there for about a year or so until the shop closed down. Maybe I was the kiss of death to all these businesses!

There were a few weeks when I did voluntary work sorting out books and cupboards at my local church, the Narrabeen Baptist church, which I quite liked as well.

So, work has always been difficult for me; I had trouble comprehending what my bosses said to me but was too inhibited to ask for clarification. I was easily bored and found it difficult to concentrate, deal with people and adapt to change. All typical problems for someone with Asperger's syndrome—if only I'd known I had it. But I was 25 before my family and I finally found out what made life such a challenge for me.

6

Not Another Doc!
Finally, A Diagnosis

Sometimes I feel like a walking list of diagnoses. I've been dragged backwards and forwards to see more doctors, therapists and specialists than I care to remember. Last count, the list was over 50. I have seen so many counsellors that I reckon I could almost run a therapy group myself.

When I was little my parents would say to me, 'Now, we've found another person to try to help us!'

My reply was, 'What! Another doctor? What for this time? Okay I'll come along with you ...'

It was always a bit of an adventure because the doctors were always so interested in me and wanted to know all about me. Adult company was good for me because I was appreciated for being me and I felt quite special. I was willing to answer anything and everything. I was eager to please and my young mind was always trying to grasp whatever the adults were talking about around me.

Some doctors would just sit in their chairs going 'Hmmm ... That's very interesting...' while I was talking away at them. Then others would give me different puzzles or tests to do that I thought was a whole load of fun. After all, I was having a day off school and wasn't getting teased or hassled for a few hours. It was boring, though, when the adults would go into a room and talk for what seemed like many hours. I'd just sit there quietly wondering what was going on in there.

First things first. I was born in the Sydney Adventist Hospital on Friday, 8 September 1972 by Caesarean section, and arrived safely. My parents especially considered me a miracle baby as they had wanted me for a very long time indeed. I was their firstborn child and the first grandchild in my family. They were very proud parents and took me home to Singleton to show off their bouncing baby girl.

When I was a year old our little family moved to Perth, Western Australia. It was around this time that my parents noticed that I wasn't like all the 'normal' babies and toddlers around. It seemed I was a little different in some ways, which really worried them.

They tell me that I had my own rather strange ways about me. For instance I seemed overly affectionate with strangers, and I would hide from mum when we were out shopping. At home I liked to line up my little toys very carefully for hours, but I wouldn't play with them like other children.

Over the years I saw speech therapists (one had me wearing a chin-cup at night to help align my jaw!), had my hearing and sight checked, and visited occupational therapists. An early childhood team who assessed me when I was seven said I had minimal brain dysfunction (MBD) and that I would grow out of it by the time I was about 10 years old.

In Sydney I was taken to see Dr Gordon Serfontein who was doing some quite interesting research into something new. ADD they called it. I was only about 10 years old at the time but I well remember one test he gave me that was slightly uncomfortable because he had to put a special gel on certain parts of my head and some type of electrodes were attached to them. All the wires in the special cap felt like a large, overgrown giant spider on my head, standing with its feet in the gel.

The test was basically to record the electronic signals and output of my brain but all I remember is that I came out of there with extremely messy and sticky hair. I don't think the doctor even gave me a treat of a lolly, yet I sure felt that I deserved one after that little episode. He prescribed Ritalin which was meant be a new magic drug. It helped me for a while, but soon the good effects became less noticeable.

Over the next few years it was a round of paediatricians and child psychologists. I also went to a food allergy centre, of all places, to try to find out if perhaps something I was eating was the cause of it all. My mum and I both had blood tests and I found out I was sensitive to tomatoes, malt, chocolate, bananas and corn. For a while I went on a special diet that excluded all those foods, and this seemed to help a little.

By this time puberty had fully hit and I was on the roller-coaster ride of the teenage years, which was not fun for anyone involved including my family, school and friends. I was a natural force of my own to be reckoned with by those around me. My demeanour was stormy, fiery, rebellious and very wild. If someone cornered me I'd be like a wildcat defending myself, claws and all.

My teenage years were filled with visits to counsellors, both Christian and non-Christian, careers counsellors and intelligence testing, as well as a couple of support and holiday groups for other troubled teens, including Dalwood at one of my worst points.

~

Having fully explored conventional medicine, after leaving high school I decided to explore more spiritual and religious views. For over a year I attended a Pentecostal church and took part enthusiastically in the various Bible studies and activities.

It was here on 5 May 1991, just one month after my traumatic first suicide attempt, that I met up again with Alex. We had known each other as children and not seen each other since. He became my first true love, and the whole experience blew me away. Suddenly life looked brighter—and possible. But more of this later.

Love, though, did not solve all my problems. Quite unexpectedly a Christian friend of my parents asked, 'Did anyone ever put a curse on you?' Was I cursed? Always keen for a solution, my parents took me to someone who was said to have a real spiritual gift for prayer therapy, unlocking repressed memories, binding demons and spirits, healing and spiritual counselling. He prayed over me, but some freaky things happened after that.

In between those times I saw a psychiatrist, a TAFE counsellor and a careers counsellor at the CES.

In 1992, when I was 20 years old, I started going back to my regular church where I was with a Bible study group and being counselled by the youth pastor. That wasn't really helping me much either so I went to another Christian counsellor, a lady in the church. By 1994 things were really coming to a head and she more than likely felt helpless to assist me.

From 1995 onwards it seemed as if I was on a very fast treadmill. I was seeing a couple of psychotherapists, a specialist in ADD, a couples' counsellor and a psychiatrist. I even saw a clinical psychologist for intelligence testing. All these and therapy groups!

In March 1996 I was admitted to another clinic where I went to the in-house patient groups and nearly all the 12-step meetings, to see what they were like, on top of seeing the psychiatrist and therapist there. I was being overloaded with all these strange new ideas where I started to doubt God yet began to refer to him as 'The Higher Power'. I felt that I was a lost cause because I was anti-medication and had virtually given up on life itself, which I hated.

I left this clinic around late-August1996, and fell headlong back into an abusive relationship, so things became a thousand times worse.

~

The answers finally started coming to us in 1998. On 1 May that year, my parents and I visited clinical psychologist Lydia Fegan, in Sydney; she changed all our lives forever. In just a couple of hours in her rooms she found that I had all the classic symptoms of Asperger's syndrome.

I was 25 years old at the time. It is much easier for children born with Asperger's today, who grow up with the right support in and out of school. I'd had so little support and understanding.

The whole family breathed a big sigh of relief after many years of not knowing what was up with me. We could now start to deal with it and treat it in its proper setting after so long. One of the reasons why I wasn't formally diagnosed until then was because it wasn't well known. An Austrian doctor, Hans Asperger, identified Asperger's syndrome as a neurobiological disorder in 1944, but it was not until 1994 that it was admitted into the Autism Spectrum of Disorders. His paper at the time described several young patients with normal intelligence who exhibited behaviour similar to people with autism.

Up until 1998 I had seen as many as 57 professionals.

~

Sometimes I think of myself as being a Miss Bean. I'm the female version of Mr Bean, living in my own small world having my own quirky little behaviours.

When I watch Mr Bean I can relate so much to him; I'm like him in real life. He does the kinds of things I do and has the ideas that I have. One example is how he locks different parts of his car and keeps his key locked in the last place he opens which is the engine so no-one would know where it was. He's very security conscious like I am and has different rituals like me. Like him, I made sure I had two sets of my car keys in case I got locked out.

In one episode Mr Bean has great trouble sleeping one night. He tries to count all the sheep he has on a poster, but still he can't sleep. So in sheer frustration he gets a calculator and counts all the sheep going downwards and then sideways ... multiplies the numbers, sees the figure and then falls straight to sleep on his bed. I often have trouble sleeping and try to do things to amuse my mind. If something's troubling me I find I just have to write it down to let it out and then I can go straight to sleep.

I do my own thing, too, walking to the beat of my own drum, usually against what is the flow for most 'normal people'. What is 'normal' anyway?

~

Another funny character who I can relate to is Basil Fawlty from *Fawlty Towers*. At the beginning of each episode he is off in his own little world doing his own thing. But in each episode there are always myriad dramas going on around him in which he ultimately becomes involved. Basil always comes out the worse for wear!

The outrageous ways he deals with all the relationships in his life and the way he always gets so worked up is ever so funny, but he's often misunderstood. I can really identify with that. I have the whole series of that show on DVD and I always end up laughing like I did when I was a kid. It cheers me up knowing that I'm not alone in my awkward experiences of life!

I often feel like an alien in this world, trying to understand a silent, garbled and very foreign language. I never seem to get it quite right, no matter how hard I try.

It feels like I am living in a diamond bubble looking outwards questioningly at everything going on around me. I feel isolated until another person with the same condition comes along and we can connect, sensing each other's feelings.

Diamonds are the hardest rocks. Nothing can scratch, cut or affect them like another diamond. So someone else with Asperger's can relate better to another person with the same condition because they are on the same wavelength and can understand one another.

I had always felt alone having Asperger's because, until 2003 when I was on holiday in Queensland and met a little boy with Asperger's syndrome, I was the only person I knew who had it. He was the first other person I had met with my condition. It was amazing to meet this boy.

I still felt lost, though, because I'd never met any adults with Asperger's. It wasn't until about 2005 when I went to an Asperger's adult social group in Sydney that I was able to meet other people who were similar to me.

Meeting people like that after travelling this world alone all my life was like a real answer to prayer for me. At last I wasn't the odd one out in this amazing galaxy of intelligent and creative people; I just have Asperger's—and there are many diamonds just like me.

7

It's Not All Bad—Asperger's Symptoms And Strengths

Asperger's Syndrome Symptoms

This is a list of Asperger's symptoms, some of which I know I have. I will give more details later on how they affect me.

- The inability to communicate properly with others
- Age-inappropriate behaviour and reactions
- Quirky little habits, rituals or ritualistic actions
- Repetitive behaviour, obsessive actions, liking repetitive sounds, music or sequences
- The inability to adjust to changes in routines
- Trouble starting new things without proper support or direction
- Loner, aloof behaviour, which can impair relating to other people
- Mostly more comfortable with studying or trying to understand people on TV, DVDs or through books
- A lack of empathy towards people
- Can take things too literally
- The inability to judge people's character properly
- Obsessive about a few subjects

- Dramatically overreact to very simple events that don't upset others
- A tendency to talk 'at' people instead of 'to' people
- Can retreat into a private little world when faced with uncomfortable or new situations
- Can come out with off-the-wall comments that can shock or surprise people
- Great trouble reading or understanding social cues
- Can have a lot of deep heavy feelings going on inside without knowing how to communicate them properly to others
- Lacking in a sense of humour. Mostly unable to understand jokes— misinterpretation of jokes
- A big tendency to keep things to oneself
- A very high or above average intelligence level with a broad range of general knowledge
- Like a big kid socially
- Things are often extremely 'black and white' or very rigid
- Not good at cause and effect
- Can quite often have a very blank or confused look in some social situations
- Trouble joining in with other people's conversations, perhaps only standing there looking at and/or listening to the other people involved in the conversation
- A tendency to use really formal, technical or elaborate language
- Hard to understand people leaving, dying, going away, not speaking anymore
- Sometimes hard to understand a point of view—it can be like talking to a brick wall
- Can be stuck in a time warp
- Can be totally disorganised
- May be vulnerable
- Can make the same mistakes over and over without learning
- Can severely misinterpret things
- Little or no understanding of time or numbers

- Can be overwhelmed by sensory and information overload and life's pressures
- Can be so focused on one thing that everything else is forgotten
- Does things in the wrong order or sequence
- Competitive and wanting to be first
- Can be very blinkered on a lot of things—walking in a minefield past signs
- Great anxiety staying in totally new places, especially overnight.

It would be a mistake to think that Aspies (for that is the friendly nickname which seems to have stuck now) are less creative and imaginative than others. In fact, Asperger's syndrome delivers a unique mix of talents and abilities.

I've discovered that it's not always everyday people who have Asperger's syndrome. Over the past 10 years or so there has been debate among researchers and other people about famous people, mostly men, who have had traits of Asperger's and autism, including Ludwig van Beethoven, Alexander Graham Bell, Wolfgang Amadeus Mozart, Isaac Newton and Hans Christian Andersen. More contemporary figures may include John Denver, Jim Henson, Alfred Hitchcock, Michael Jackson, Andy Kaufman and Andy Warhol.

Jane Austen, Cleopatra and Catherine the Great are among the small number of women throughout history thought to have had Asperger's. As history shows us, not many women have this condition so it's important for us females who do have it to show that we can stand up for ourselves.

There have also been a few television characters such as Bert on *Sesame Street*, Basil Fawlty from *Fawlty Towers* and the well-known Mr Bean who have shown traits of Asperger's and autism.

Although Aspies see the world in a different way, and may have difficulties interacting in a social context, life is still a positive experience. I will share just a few insights to demonstrate this.

Asperger's Traits That Can Be Strengths For Me

1. Determination: I don't give up on things; I'm like a dog with a bone!
2. Single-mindedness: when's something's in my head I go for it
3. Black and white thinking: very strict about right and wrong
4. Inability to lie
5. Very good memory: music, movies, general knowledge and facts
6. Very high intelligence: I can understand a lot of things in an intelligent, creative way
7. Enjoy routines: once in a routine I'm often very, very comfortable and function a whole lot better. I'm less anxious or scared when I know what's going on
8. Good visual and spatial awareness: I have a really good sense of direction but often can't remember street names; I'm very good at remembering pictures and photographs and people's faces
9. Very loyal: in a relationship I don't give up and often think of ways of improving it if it's bad or having troubles; I stick by my friends and family no matter what
10. Very thorough and pedantic: even though I am slow, I make sure things are just right
11. Technical ability: I always read the instructions and follow them to a 'T'.

~

The following are day-to-day examples of how my Asperger's symptoms have served as strengths for me.

Brookvale, 1990

When I was working in electronics assembly something interesting happened. Whether it was from the solder fumes, a hangover, or a virus, I suddenly collapsed one day and was taken to the medical centre and then hospital. I had pain in both my head and my body. The young woman doctor couldn't work out what was wrong with me. As she was poking and prodding me she was asking me questions.

'Now Megan, do you know where you are?'

'Yes. I'm at Manly Hospital,' was my reply.

She continued, 'What day of the week is it?'

'Tuesday of course,' was my reply.

I didn't know why she was asking me all these questions and I felt strange about it. Yet a few more questions came along which I answered correctly. Then the last one: 'Now Megan. Can you tell me what the capital of Iceland is?'

'Yes. The capital is Reykjavik. I can even try to spell it for you if you want!' I replied promptly.

There was a stunned silence in the room. The doctor stopped examining me for a moment, looked at me and then said, 'Do you realise you are the first patient ever in my life to get that question right? I'm amazed at your knowledge!'

I looked at her in surprise and said, ' Really? Really, am I the first patient to get that?'

The doctor replied with a smile, 'Yes you are! I normally throw that in as a brainteaser and don't expect anyone to get it right, because it's not a well-known place.'

The nurse said with a big smile, 'Well done, Megs! I didn't even know the answer for that! You're full of surprises.'

The examination finished and my instructions were to rest until I felt better, which was fine with me.

My good general knowledge has come in handy over the years when watching TV quiz shows with my family after dinner; I would get a lot of the answers right. Both my parents have suggested over the years, 'Hey, Megs! You should try to go on one of those shows. You'll blitz them and could win yourself a whole lot of money!'

'Yeah, thanks guys, I think I'll give it a try,' was always my reply.

I called the comp lines of *Who Wants To Be A Millionaire?* once, but I didn't get in. I just love learning facts about different things. I also like to surprise someone in a conversation with a bit of trivia or a little-known fact. I like seeing people's faces when I say something a bit offbeat and off the wall!

Learning opens up more of this world for me. It helps me to understand what's going on a whole lot better, which is good. Sure there are subjects I have no idea about, for whatever reason, but I tend to really focus on the ones I love, which is typical for Asperger's. Some people talk about the 'little professor' quirk which some Aspies have—they may begin a conversation with a little-known fact or use large and learned words in general conversation.

However, my good general knowledge doesn't help me with my social skills. But that's life and as long as you're happy, that's the main thing.

Brookvale, 2007

It was late Wednesday afternoon when my girlfriend at the time dropped her teenage son off to his trumpet lesson. We were sitting in the car and didn't want to wait for ages. Looking across at me she said, 'Hey, Megs, how about we go for a walk up the street for a bit?'

'That sounds like a good idea!' I replied with a glint in my eye.

So we started to walk along the tree-lined streets in the beautiful afterglow of the sun as it slowly went down. Having 'Us' time together, going for a walk and sharing things after a busy day, was important for us to chill out. On our walk we discovered a park and we sat down on a bench. Something caught my attention.

In the far corner of the park I noticed a pair of swings and another piece of playground equipment that I found extremely inviting. I was getting a bit distracted, remembering having fun on the swings as a kid. I looked at my girlfriend beside me, then at the swings … then back at her again.

'Hey babe! Do you wanna go for a ride on the swings over there?' I said with a big cheeky smile on my face.

She had a really perplexed look and asked, 'Really! A ride on the swings? I can't remember when I last did it! I'm not sure …'

'C'mon it'll be fun, babe! It lets your inner child out. It's good to do!' I said encouragingly. She was still looking at me quizzically and I gave her a quick kiss on the cheek. Suddenly she said, 'Okay! Let's go for a swing!'

We linked arms and started walking down to the swings. We saw two other people come into the park, which made her feel uncomfortable, so we unlinked our arms. She was always nervous about PDAs (public displays of affection), which I found a bit hard sometimes.

When I got on the swing and began swinging it felt like I was a child again. Almost. Then, going for a swing was the most important thing in the world and all your troubles flew away on wings and prayers. It was like a freeing experience and, looking over at my girlfriend, I noticed a beautiful smile on her face. She was relaxed and at ease in her own way and I loved to see that side of her.

'Megs, I'm having fun here!' she said swinging past me. My swing was getting higher and faster and as I swung past her I raised my voice and cried, 'That's so great to hear, babe! It means a lot to me!'

With the cool air around us it was almost like we were two little girls again sharing a few innocent moments on the swing together. We slowly stopped our swinging, sitting there feeling really relaxed. We looked at each other and she winked at me with her cute smile and I at her. Our thoughts turned back to walking to the car and waiting for her son to finish his lesson. The cool darkness of the evening was starting to surround us but our hearts were brimming with pure affection for one another. We got back in the car and its warmth was comforting. I put my hand on hers, our hands slowly warming each other up. We both sat there in a total silence where no words were needed, simply sharing the moment together.

Sharing the experience of being a kid in an adult's body with her meant so much to me. It was like sharing a bit of the heavenly innocence of childhood again where we are all free to be who we want to be, having fun, playing. All through my life it's always been extremely important to reconnect to the pure joy and enthusiasm of being a child. It always remains important to me and I hope I never lose it.

USA, 1990

'Holidays here we come. The Hammond family is hitting the world!' I shouted.

For months the whole family had been saving carefully. My parents had had a few troubles with their teenage kids, more so with me. At the time I was really rough around the edges and extremely rebellious. I had actually been retrenched from my job not long before we were to leave, so I knew I had no job to come back to.

But all of this didn't matter as we stepped on the plane. What lay before us was several weeks of an unforgettable family holiday with dramas, fun and an amazing country as the backdrop. We had never been to America before but dad had lived there as a small kid for a while.

Our main destination was Minneapolis, Minnesota, which was still many hours away with a couple of plane rides to reach it. Here some very dear friends of the family met us tired and weary Aussie travellers. For the next week our family was going to see the corn-growing heartland of America and the Minnesota state fair, which was the place to go.

One hot day our friends took us to one of the lakes. It was a perfect day for waterskiing. Uncle Lowell rigged the boat up on the trailer. My brother Cameron was so excited and asked, 'Hey, dad, are we going waterskiing today?'

'Yes, son, we are at last going. So you can now try to do it!' dad said with a huge smile on his face. Dad, being the adventurous soul that he is, of course could do it, but none of us others could.

'Let's go waterskiing, old mate!' Uncle Lowell said in his broad American accent with a watermelon smile to match.

So the two biggest kids of them all went in the water first and showed off. Then came my brother's turn and they rigged up the beginners' boom bar for him. After only a few tries he managed to get upright, which was amazing because he'd never done it before.

'Hey, you guys, I can ski! I can do it! I'm standing!' he cried out with a shaky smile.

Everyone in the boat cheered. He graduated to skiing behind

the boat, which was another huge achievement for a first-timer. Then Uncle Lowell turned to me and said, 'Now, Megs, it's your turn to try it!'

'It sure is! I'm sure I can do it!' I said with adrenaline rushing through my whole body and very inspired by the others.

So I put my life jacket on, jumped off the side of the boat near the special bar, put my skis on and yelled out, 'I'm ready, let's go waterskiing!'

Little did I know what was ahead! The first time I was shaky and fell back in, then watched the boat do a U-turn to get to me again. Words of encouragement were coming from the boat as I put on my skis again. The second time I felt like I was going to get it, but fell down again splashing in the water. The next time dad and Uncle Lowell both chimed in with tips: ' What you do, Megs, is pretend you're sitting down in the water and hold the pose until the boat pulls you up! Before you know it you'll be standing like the rest of us!'

'Sure, I'll give it a try. Thank you for that. I'll do it,' I chimed back.

As I sat in the water I was so determined, I was psyching myself up for it completely. I thought to myself, okay, it's third time lucky. I can do this. I know I can!

The boat started to pull me forward and I was improving a bit, but at the last minute I fell in the water again. Attempt number four and I was starting to feel a bit tired. The boat revved up and started to pull me forward, but I hit the water yet again. The next couple of times were forgettable but mum and Aunty Kathy kept up the cheering.

I thought to myself, I am not getting out of this lake until I can eventually stand up like all the others did. I am not going to give up on this! I got myself along the side of the boat and Cameron had a cheeky smile on his face.

Uncle Lowell said, 'Let's try again, Megs! We all know that you will do it!'

The seventh attempt you'd think would be lucky and I'd be standing up like a pro wouldn't you? But I ended up in the water again to my surprise, even after so many times. After a few more times my legs were jelly and my body betrayed me; it decided that enough was enough after 11 or so valiant tries. I was even too tired to climb back into the boat.

That night Aunty Kathy said proudly, ' I have never ever seen anyone try so hard to learn how to ski, without giving up. You've impressed me you have, Megs.'

'Thanks, Aunty Kathy. I really do appreciate it. My mind and spirit was willing but my body wasn't, unfortunately,' I replied.

The next day I woke up and I was as stiff as a board from top to toe. I felt a huge sense of achievement, even though I didn't get up on the skis.

Throughout my life I've discovered that I have a very rare gift of determination and do not give up on things that are close to my heart.

Brookvale, 2001

One day all the buzzers were going crazy on the wards of a clinic in Cremorne where I had been admitted a week before. A lot were just buzzing at random times, others didn't seem to be working properly. I saw a couple of electrical workers scurrying throughout the building and then the face of a lady. Instantly, it was like a bolt of lightning went through my chest. I knew I recognised her from somewhere. I walked off to have a think and then said to myself, 'Aha! Hey, she used to work with me back in 1990!'

So I went back to the level she was working on and although I felt really nervous I had to go up to find out whether it was her or not. I approached her and asked, 'Excuse me? Does your name happen to be Barbara?'

She stopped what she was doing and looked at me, amused, before answering in her Polish accent, 'Yes my name's Barbara. Now where do I know you from?'

'My name's Megan! Do you remember me? We worked together about 11 years ago. I only worked there for a few months.'

A flicker of recognition came over her face and then the hint of a smile and she said, 'Yes, I think I may remember you now. You have an extremely good memory there!'

So we ended up standing there talking and catching up for a few minutes and then wished each other luck and went our separate ways again. Because I have such an excellent memory for people's faces my mother says I should have become a detective—or maybe an immigration officer! I've recognised people up to 20 years after I've last seen them, much to the astonishment of the people involved.

Even though my memory is excellent my people skills are still almost naive in a lot of ways. Just recently at church I saw a lady in her 60s who I hadn't seen since I was a teenager. I asked a friend of mine who was with me, 'What's Kira doing here?'

Val simply replied, 'Why don't you go ask her.'

So I walked up to Kira and the first words that came out of my mouth, after 20 years, were, 'Hey, Kira, what are you doing here?'

She looked at me, a bit taken aback, and then I continued, 'Do you remember me? I'm Megan Hammond. Do you remember me, from many years ago?'

Val was behind me and was maybe trying to help remind her by mouthing something. Kira's face changed a bit and she said, 'Hammond? Okay! I've started coming back here again after many years. Good to see you.'

Then she started talking to someone else. It wasn't long after that I realised the way I spoke to her was a bit strange and maybe even rude. Who in their right mind would go up to someone they hadn't seen in 20 years and ask them what they were doing in church?

Being abrupt to others is a typical Asperger's thing. But when I recognise a face I feel like it is almost a gift to remember them as a person at whatever stage they were at in their lives when I knew them. I never know who I'm going to bump into when I walk out the door. Remembering people's faces is a valuable skill and makes life very interesting!

Brookvale, 1999

I find I often have to tell the truth no matter what the cost is for me. Honesty and integrity are of the highest importance for me.

I remember one night in my early 20s, when I attended an important function with my parents and many of mum's work colleagues. My brother and I had to be on our best behaviour. I felt like drinking, however, and throughout the evening my behaviour worsened as I got drunk. At the end we all caught the elevator to street level. When we got into the car my parents, Cameron and his friend were angry with me because of how I had behaved.

'Stuff this! I'm going to find some more drinks to have somewhere else!' I said getting out of the car and starting to walk off.

The window came down and dad tooted the horn while mum called out, 'Come back and get in the car, Megs! You're not in a safe state of mind!'

Looking back at them I blurted out, 'I don't think so, guys! I'm sick of it!' and walked off quickly.

So, late at night and very drunk, I wandered the streets of the city. I saw a supermarket on a corner so I thought I'd walk through there to see what it was like. It was quite busy and I saw a cheap, black pair of sunglasses that took my fancy. The feel and the look of the sunglasses really appealed to me for some strange reason. Next thing, I'd stowed them in my bag and quickly walked out of the shop. To my surprise when I got out on the street no-one from the store followed me. I was in a state of shock because I'd never stolen anything from a shop before.

The next thought that came into my head was, 'Hey! How about I walk up Oxford Street to see what's open at this time of night?'

So I found myself walking up to the Burdekin Hotel, almost on automatic pilot, because the alcohol was clouding my judgement. The pub was fairly quiet and I tried to walk up to the bar as soberly as I could to order a drink of spirits. I found somewhere to sit and drown my sorrows with a few more drinks and some borrowed cigarettes from people near me. Not long after that I was cut off from the bar so I walked up the road to find another pub.

I ordered a drink, sat down and talked to a woman near me who was drinking also. I ended up walking her to her unit block where she left me downstairs. Come to think of it, I was probably annoying her without realising it. I walked down the street for quite a bit and caught a taxi home feeling really the worse for wear.

The next day I was sick with the worst hangover and found the sunglasses with the tag still on them in my bag. As soon as I saw them my heart sank with immense guilt.

Over the next few days I decided that I had to face up to the consequences of stealing something. So I caught a bus back into the city, walked up to the counter attendant in the supermarket, gave her back the sunglasses and said something like, 'Hello there! About a week ago I was really drunk and I was in this shop. I saw these sunglasses and stole them … Don't worry, I haven't used them and I thought I'd be honest and give them back because I couldn't live with what I had done. Thank you!'

The lady's face was priceless: shock and surprise mingled with bewilderment. All she could stutter was something like, 'Thank you for giving them back!'

No more was said between us and I walked out of the store with a huge weight lifted from my soul!

There have been plenty of other times where I've been too honest for my own good, but I see it as a strength that keeps me in line. It is part of who I am as a person, and I have Asperger's to thank for it.

8

How Asperger's Has Affected Me

All through my life people have said that I'm a bit odd—strange, weird, a square peg trying to fit into a round hole, mad, psycho, crazy, out of left field, eccentric, an enigma, a mystery, a curse, a blessing, a bird in the wrong nest, a bit out there—among a whole lot of other things.

Many misunderstand me—but I can hardly blame them. Let's face it; I am only just beginning to understand myself!

Like many people with Asperger's I tend to take things quite literally. For this reason I often don't get the point of jokes and people sometimes get angry with me as they don't want to spoil things by explaining the punch line to me. This really annoys me as I want to understand why they are laughing and be part of it.

A lot of my quirks and habits are ways of relieving my anxiety and trying to put some order into my world; they take me away from reality and give me comfort. Another thing I share with other Aspies is fixations on objects or people. As a baby the toy of choice for me to sleep with was a red horseshoe magnet, which I was greatly attached to, and later a toy called Froggy.

As a small child I was also fascinated by a photo of a friend of my parents' in their college yearbook. From a sea of faces there she was looking out at me, and I rarely let the book out of my sight. She, like my magnet, became my constant companion.

Sadly these fixed ideas were often strange or negative and my obsessions baffled everyone around me, including myself.

The following are examples of how Asperger's has affected me during my life and show how vulnerable and stressed I can be when it comes to change and hardship, relationships and people in general.

Dealing With Change, Kalgoorlie, 1981

'Kids! Come inside please. Mum and I have something to tell you,' dad's voice came from the back porch.

My brother and I stopped playing, looking at each other puzzled. We both yelled out in unison, 'Yes, dad, we're coming!'

We stopped playing in our grassy backyard; grass was quite unusual in Kalgoorlie because the town is situated on the edge of the desert in Western Australia. We ran into our huge federation house and sat ourselves down on the lounge, waiting expectantly for the news. Dad said, 'Now, kids, we have something to tell you that's important.'

There was a strange silence and he continued, 'Kids, it looks like we have to move to Sydney with my work quite soon.'

You could hear a pin drop in the room for a second. Then I heard my brother's voice saying, 'Why, dad? We like it here in Kalgoorlie; it's so much fun.'

I chimed in. 'We're not going to be away forever are we? What about all our friends who live here? I like living here!'

We both looked pleadingly at my parents for answers that they couldn't give us. Finally dad tried to reassure us by saying, 'Look, kids, we're only going to be over there for about four or five years and it's more than likely we are going to come back here.'

That didn't sit right in my nine-year-old head. I had trouble calculating how old I was going to be when we came back. Cameron, who was younger, was maybe a bit more positive about it than I was. Mum and dad gave us both a great big hug trying to comfort us; great changes were afoot for us as a family.

Over the next couple of months our family slowly packed the house up and made preparations to leave our friends. All these things happening felt quite surreal to me, but we were going to see my grandparents over in Sydney, which was good.

Before us was the trip of a lifetime crossing the Nullarbor Plain. It must have been a huge test of patience for our parents having two kids prone to fighting in a confined space for 2000 odd kilometres. But they made it as much fun as possible and we listened to tapes and played car games along the way.

Finally we made it to Sydney where we all had to unpack everything again. The house was a whole lot smaller than the one in Kalgoorlie. It was then that it hit me in a big way that Western Australia, my home state, was behind me and everything was brand new, which I disliked with a passion. My bedroom was different, my school was no longer there, I had no friends, I had to go to a different school and church, I had to find a new occupational therapist and speech therapist.

My whole life was turned upside down and my head was spinning with confusion. I cried almost every night to my parents, pleading with them to take me back to Kalgoorlie, but to no avail. The homesickness that I felt was gutting me to the point that I couldn't sleep properly. Instead I found myself reading books in my bed from about 1am for many hours. The books were my friends and my escape; I could lose myself in them. One of the only things I liked was seeing my grandparents and other cousins more often. Sydney was like a strange foreign country to me where everyone was different.

Moving to Sydney was like a huge kick in the pants and I believed my life would never be the same again from that day forward.

I still find change difficult. Recently two friends asked me, 'How's it going? Do you want to come out for a few hours to catch up?' Then they suggested I stay over and mind their small yappy dog for a week because they had a wedding to go to in Goulburn.

Well, that night was the start of a nightmare week for someone living and coping with Asperger's. The new surroundings and environment, new people and different routines totally threw me. I felt like a duck out of water, trying to hold decent conversations with people I didn't know, trying to explain things to them, sleeping (or rather not sleeping) in a different bed, eating different food, cars breaking down then catching public transport, which I wasn't used to.

Like most people with Asperger's I just don't cope with change at all well. By that Friday night I was totally exhausted.

Finally free of my dog-minding duties, I visited my girlfriend, expecting to be there only for an hour or so. Unexpectedly I had a total meltdown; my mind stopped thinking, understanding or comprehending things around me. I felt like a lead balloon had fallen on me and was pushing me far underground and I was stuck there. What was worse was that I was shaking like a leaf and having flashbacks from the post-traumatic stress brought on by a former partner's treatment of me.

I felt so terrible because my girlfriend had to witness me go through stuff I normally battle alone and don't show anyone. The poor woman must have thought I was going half-crazy but my body, mind and emotions went on automatic shutdown; in no way could I help it. It took several days to recover from that unexpected week and its effect on me.

I put every ounce of my energy, day after day, into trying to deal with things that normal people find easy.

Having Asperger's can be exhausting.

An Ordered, Disordered World, Sydney, 1981 onwards

Sitting on buses to and from school I was armed with pens, pencil and a notebook or pad of paper. I found it important to write down all the information and things I saw around me. First at the top of the pad I felt I had to write what date it was, not once, but in a few different ways: 29/6/81 Monday, 29 June 1981, 29-Jun-81, 29/6/81 8.27:55am.

To be exact was very important to me. I also wrote down the numbers of interesting registration plates I saw and liked, such as DAM 236 or RAT 777. I liked ones that made words. Or I'd play with the words of the sign 'Signal Driver' at bus stops. I'd write words like 'sign', 'drive' or 'river', or other things made out of those words.

One afternoon a schoolmate on the bus asked me, 'Hey Megs, what would you rather be called as a name?'

I replied that I would rather be called Frances or Lea and this provoked laughter. As I tried to explain why I like those names so much the laughter got louder and more raucous. By then all the other passengers were starting to look up at the back of the bus. That was another afternoon ritual where I'd be sitting quietly and sometimes the other kids from my school would begin to make fun of me.

I didn't want to be associated with the immature mob of schoolkids on the bus so I retreated into my own little world of looking out for different numberplates and writing different words and names down. I also liked making up and inventing my own unique names like Zoltan, Zoltar, Xenos, Zoftahaha. Or I'd play on the different spellings of names like 'Lee' as in Lei, Lea, Lie, Leah, Le and all the derivations of them. The more strange the name, the more I liked it.

Sydney, 1982

You could say that for much of my childhood I inhabited my own little world, which was more comfortable for me. Order was important, and having special items around me was vital.

For instance, when we moved from Western Australia, I decided to pack my large rock collection. I wrapped each rock in tissues or newspaper, securing it with sticky tape. I think I took more care of my rocks than anything else that I had to pack. It was imperative because they were part of me and the Kalgoorlie I loved. Upon arrival in this new and very different state, I eagerly unpacked my box of rocks. At last I was reunited with some of my old friends, which was a real comfort to me.

'Froggy! Froggy! Where's my froggy? I NEED my froggy! Mum?' These words gushed out of me as fast as the anxiety was coming into my body.

There was no answer at all and I was left in this prison of emotion.

'My froggy! He's the only friend that I have left! What am I going to do? I'm so lost! Where's mum?' I thought to myself.

'Mum! I need my little froggy! Please help me?' I bleated out more softly this time, for this little lamb felt so lost.

Next thing I heard was mum joining me in my room. 'Sorry, Megs, I was just getting dressed and ready for Sabbath School. You've lost your froggy have you?' She leant down and gave me a comforting hug that only a mother could give.

Within an instant she found Froggy and then she helped me dress.

Froggy was my constant companion and only friend at that difficult time. He was my biggest comfort since moving to Sydney. During those first years Froggy and I were inseparable. He came to school with me and sat in front of me on my desk and I also slept with him in my bed. He was almost alive and over the years he got very raggedy, like 'The Velveteen Rabbit'; he lost an eye and also got a hole in one of his feet where the stuffing slowly disappeared from him, like grains of sand.

I loved Froggy for he was my only friend on Earth who seemed to love and accept me with no judgements. Froggy, my Froggy, I'll never forget you my dear friend!

Sydney, 1982 onwards

Like most kids I loved lots of hugs and affection from people around me. I loved connecting to people on that level and it made me feel really nice and warm inside. My mum and I would be walking in public in a shopping centre somewhere and she would be looking at something interesting in the shop window. Suddenly for some reason I needed a hug from her so I would ask, 'Hey mum, can I please have a hug because I feel like one?'

Mum would stop what she was doing, look at me and say, 'Megan, we are in a shopping centre and it's an inappropriate place for a hug. Do you understand?'

I'd shake my head slowly saying, 'No mum, I don't really understand.'

At that instant I felt like I was a few centimetres tall. I had no understanding at all of what she meant.

It seemed I had no idea of the right times for asking for hugs from people, which I found hard. One day mum was preparing food in the kitchen and she had flour all over her hands. I just walked in asking for a hug and she stopped cooking, showing me she had food everywhere on her. 'Megs!' she said in a frustrated tone. 'Not now! It's the wrong timing! I've got food everywhere and my hands are dirty!' I was surprised so I just stuttered, 'Um … um … I'm sorry, mum, I didn't realise!' Then I walked out of the room in great embarrassment.

When I was very small I would hug people who I had just met, or take an instant liking to someone and hang around them all the time, much to my parents' worry and embarrassment.

When I was older and used to get drunk a lot I became really different and even more affectionate; I'd hug total strangers and be very friendly with them. I've had a few friends, Beck and Justine, who have worried about me over the years for being over-affectionate with people. They'd often pull me aside and tell me to back off because it could give people the wrong impression about me. Drinking could be disastrous for me. That's the main reason I hardly drink anymore.

I guess with my upbringing and my condition I think that people are the same as me—having been brought up with morals, ethics and guidelines to live a better life—when they are not. Also, having Asperger's makes it difficult for me to see things through other people's eyes.

I can have very black and white views also, and have quite strict ideas about different things. I've been told that in non-Christian circles or bar-drinking circles, if you give a guy a hug then it is a come-on or a lead-up to having sex. Even today I often stuff up when it comes to appropriate times for hugs and other social etiquette. I still have great trouble understanding body contact rules, but I'm a whole lot better than I once was.

Dee Why, 1982 onwards

Frustration zapped through my 10-year-old body. My mind was on overload. Impulsively I put my hands out in front of my body and started karate chopping them into the air, very fast. I don't know why I started doing it but it seemed to give me some relief, which I needed at the time. It must have appeared very odd or weird to other people around me also. It fast grew into such a habit that eventually my parents noticed. One day mum caught sight of me doing it. She stopped short and asked, 'Megan, what are you doing? Why are you doing it?'

Her stunned look said it all, but I thought nothing of it. I thought it was normal and all kids did that sort of thing. So there I was quite often doing my unique hand-flap dance. When I flapped my hands I was in a comforting world of my own where the rhythm of my hands was almost a little symphony within itself.

I also hummed to myself when I was trying to calm down. It was a way to let out the tension appropriately when I had no other healthy way to do so. Praise God that I wasn't one of these kids who hit others.

I rarely do it today but I still remember the exciting surge of adrenaline running though my arms when trying to deal with my frustrations or excitement.

Dee Why, 1983

One day, one very ordinary day, something happened. I can't remember any details of date, time or place, yet the only way I can describe it is like this ... it just happened. Something clicked deep inside me in the very back of my unconscious mind without me realising it. I don't know what the trigger was and all this is still a mystery to me and my family. It changed the entire landscape of the old relationship which my dad and I had enjoyed.

For some crazy reason I suddenly didn't want anything to do with dad; I wouldn't sit near him and even hated referring to him as 'we' in a sentence or being associated with him in any way.

It was a real mystery to everyone why I felt like that and behaved that way, because he had always been a kind and loving father to me. Being on the receiving end must have hurt him so much because there was a time before that when I was 'Daddy's little girl' and we were best friends!

Because it happened so soon after the traumatic move from Western Australia, my mum thought that maybe I was somehow blaming dad for it. But over the coming years nothing changed, although I had a similar irrational reaction to Mrs Brighteyes, my school teacher in 1984, whose sole sin was her singing voice! I was not very sensible in my reasoning.

I didn't start to warm to dad again until I was about 22 and it remains a huge mystery as to why it ever happened.

Asperger's is like that. For whatever reason, it creates mysterious behaviour, confusing even the Aspie!

Dealing With Rejection—Lane Cove, 1994

I always put my heart and soul into work because I was brought up that way. I have been taught to work to the best of my ability no matter what is thrown at me.

When I had a lunchtime car accident in 1994 I had to take time off work on workers' compensation. During that time my insurance money came back and dad found me a second-hand car, which I would need when I returned to work. I wanted to get back to work so I came up with the not-so-brilliant idea of telling the doctor I was better, then silently putting up with the pain without letting anyone know.

I reported to my supervisor, who promptly gave me something to do so I could get into the swing of it again. A short time later someone came to my desk with a message: 'Megan Hammond, can you report to the personnel office please?'

I remember thinking, 'Oh they must want to welcome me back and complete another form or something.'

I was warmly welcomed into the boss's office with a smile and a 'Hello there! Sit down!' After talking for a bit, the bullet came: 'Megan, I'm afraid that we have to let you go. Your contract's up, blah, blah, blah ...' I was hit in the heart and the words following were not sinking into my head. I felt a couple of warm tears come to my eyes and asked them why.

The answers were given but I had been so crushed beyond belief that I was flatter than a pancake. In my spacey dreamed-out fog of shock I left the office and managed to get into my car. I stopped for a minute, then started driving, driving for the sake of driving, going somewhere, not particularly going anywhere, because of my lost state.

Soon I found myself driving on the Hume Highway through the different southern suburbs and I just kept on going, going and going until I was past the outer limits of Sydney and later, the turn-off for Canberra. It seemed it wasn't me who was in control. The autopilot in my head had taken over and the driving seemed to calm me a little, in a sense giving some control over my emotions. I wanted to keep on driving and escape from everything that had happened to me in my life over the past year.

When I passed the Dog on the Tuckerbox near Gundagai, I thought to myself, I know what I'll do ... I'll go and see some friends who live in Albury as a surprise. Or I could even go on down to Melbourne to surprise my Uncle Col, if I can find him!

As it turned out I couldn't remember where any of them lived because I was in such a confused state, so I had a pit stop at a service station when I arrived in Melbourne to pick up some much needed supplies. I bought a couple of maps of Victoria, a map of Australia, a Melbourne street directory, lollies, a drink and other essentials. I wanted to go back via Geelong where I had been on a family trip once before.

Setting off from the city was quite easy, but somewhere I took the wrong turn-off, and then decided to go to Bendigo or Ballarat instead. I could have backtracked but by then it was well and truly night-time. Driving on the dark country roads made it more mystical, especially later. Somehow I did make it to Bendigo and stopped at a late-night service station. I filled up with petrol and bought a map of Bendigo, a couple of other maps and something to eat and drink. By this time I had driven many hours without proper breaks; however, I was still wide awake and full of nervous tension—pure energy running through my body.

Then I came up with another bright idea: I could go and visit Mildura where our family had a short holiday quite a few years ago.

Leaving Bendigo in a cloud of dust I started driving towards Mildura, with no clear idea of how far it was except that it was in Victoria somewhere. So I followed the signs and by this time it was really early the next morning and my car was slowly running out of petrol again, with no service station in sight. I slowed down to use less petrol. I finally stopped in a really tiny town that had no service stations open at this time in the morning. I found a phone booth and gave the RACV a call saying that I had run out of petrol and needed some assistance to get more. I rang my friend Karlyn because I needed to talk to her but hung up at the last minute because I was so scared.

Finally a very tired RACV man came with his van to assist me with a relatively small can of petrol. I think it took a while for him to rouse up from his comfortable slumber. After all, it was about 3.30 in the morning! He filled the car up with petrol then turned around and asked me to pay for it. At this point my heart sank and I informed him that I had no cash on me, but if he had EFTPOS I could then pay for it. He wasn't happy but gave me a receipt with the address to send the money to when I got back to Sydney. I thanked him profusely for rescuing me so early in the morning. We said our goodbyes, and I continued driving to Mildura.

As I was driving the tiredness was really starting to hit me but I was determined to make it to my destination. The dawn was coming and I could see kangaroos hopping along in the bush and fields around me: I'd have to be very careful of these beautiful creatures and of my car!

At this time in the morning there was hardly any traffic. Up ahead I saw the lights of a really welcoming open, yes open, service station. I immediately pulled in to get some petrol. That tired RACV man had only given me enough to get me to the next biggest and closest servo. I stocked up with some more lollies and a drink because my supplies were running so low.

Making it to Mildura was a real high point for me. I think I was trying to rediscover the happy times that we had spent together as a family on holidays. It almost felt that my family was travelling along with me on the drive as well, which made it less lonely I suppose. What I hadn't considered was that at this moment my parents were wondering where I was and were extremely worried.

After I turned the car towards Sydney I took another detour to Blayney and after 30 hours of driving I finally called my parents to let them know what was happening. I dialled the number and it rang, rang and rang more and mum answered at last, 'Hello! Who is this?'

At this point I was really hesitant to answer but I said, 'It's Megan here. I'm sorry to call like this but I wanted to let you know what was happening.'

'Where are you, Megan?' came her surprised voice on the phone, 'We have been so worried about you!'

I knew at this point I had to tell the truth with what was happening. 'Um! I'm in Bathurst. I am on my way back from Melbourne.'

For a minute there was total shocked, surprised silence on the end of the phone. You could have heard a pin drop.

'Maybe they've fainted over there!' I thought to myself.

Next came the question, 'Why on earth are you there? Bathurst is not on the way back from Melbourne!'

'Umm! Um! It is, mum, if you drive through Mildura!'

There was silence on the other end—what could she say to that!

I certainly did christen my car by taking it on such a long journey but you'd have to agree that this was an extreme reaction to being 'let go' from work. People with Asperger's and ADD, like me, often act impulsively and with intense emotion that is over the top.

Over the next 10 years or more I was going to take myself on a few more massive driving trips where I would feel free and independent. But these ones were pretty well planned and yes, those times all my family and friends knew what was happening and I kept in regular contact with them.

Standing Up For My Rights, RSL Club, 2008

Not all people with Asperger's have a speech impediment, of course, but many do have problems with language and talking.

I remember as a small child wanting to say so much yet I had no real way of communicating it. That frustrated me enormously. I didn't start talking properly until I was about four years old, which desperately worried my parents.

Recently I was helping a friend of mine, Jackie, and her family move her things back to her parents' house. After a day of moving, trying to deal with her two-month-old baby and the rainy weather, we decided to go out for a bit. Our task was to pick up some cold items from the unit she was moving from but we got a little sidetracked and went to an RSL club on the way. We entered the club in search of a quiet area to sit. Jackie bought a schooner of beer for herself and a middy for me, which we promptly downed while smoking a couple of cigarettes.

We talked about everything, ordered a couple more drinks and then it was my shout, so I walked inside and gave my order. 'Can I please have a schooner and a middy of beer, please?'

No sooner had I said that than the barman said, 'I'm sorry you've been cut off. No can do.'

I stopped short, thinking to myself, 'No way! This is so unfair. I've only had two small drinks.'

I looked at him and said, 'This can't be. It's a misunderstanding. I'm sober!'

He said, 'You have 15 minutes to leave the premises after this warning.'

I looked him straight in the eye. The barman then said 'I'm sorry! There have been reports that you've had too much to drink. You still have 15 minutes to leave. No, you can't ask another bartender, but you can talk to a supervisor if he's around ...'

I knew that I was right and I was determined to get this misunderstanding sorted out somehow because it seemed so very unfair. I had been through this sort of thing before.

When the supervisor came up, I said to him, 'I have had a speech impediment all my life and I often speak unclearly. I've only had two drinks while being here. I have a disability!'

The supervisor looked at me disbelievingly, not even batting an eyelid, then said, 'You have a disability? Do you have anything that can prove that you do actually have a disability?'

At this point I felt that I was being discriminated against so I pulled out my pension card from my wallet and handed it to him to look at it. I found that really hard because I hate showing my pension card to just any person if I can avoid it, or saying to a complete stranger that I actually have a disability. It's not like I get time off from it, like a nine-to-five job with breaks. I have this bloody condition 24 hours a day, seven days a week. I can't change what I have, but I've learned how to deal with it over the years.

I went on explaining to him and he eventually said that we could have one last drink, then leave after that. I told him that we were planning to do that anyway. He also said that it was hard from the club's side when this type of thing happened. After all this kerfuffle I was wondering what Jackie was thinking or if she was worried about me. On walking back to her outside, I felt this strong feeling of annoyance, discrimination, helplessness, frustration—but also empowerment because I had I stood up for myself.

At the end of the night I felt good because I had stood up for the truth, what I believed in and all the other people like me who have been discriminated against.

When I told my parents about it my mother, who used to work for the Spastic Centre, said people with cerebral palsy had this sort of thing happen to them when they went out to pubs and clubs. The staff, hearing their speech and seeing uncoordinated movements, thought they were drunk and refused to serve them, not really realising or understanding their condition.

So that night in the club I wasn't just standing up for me but for all those others who have been in my position. I was a small voice for the rest of the community who are just a little bit different, but still should be valued members of this world we live in.

Depression And Anxiety

Any lifetime disability attracts other issues. In the case of Asperger's, the pressures society puts on all individuals to appear 'normal' are especially taxing for people with this condition. Various emotional responses can become more serious issues, even triggering psychological ailments, and lives can spin out of control. Sometimes other things—loss, death, world events— can affect them also, complicating life even further.

I have lost so many weeks, days, even years of my life because of the black hand of depression holding me in its claws. It is like deep night totally surrounding me. Life passes me by, and I am lost in a time warp. Life stands still. I am trapped, frozen within myself.

Depression is a word that is used so widely these days and means so many different things. People can have everything from mild depression up to severe clinical depression where they are incapable of doing hardly anything. Some aren't even aware that they have symptoms of depression or are in total denial about it. Sometimes it can be masked by different actions as well.

My personal struggle with depression has been a bloody hard, challenging road that at times has seemed to have no end in sight. Depression for me has been a really black heavy cloud that weighs me down so much, to the point where my life becomes static ... still ... immovable. It has only been recently that I've realised the full extent that depression has got in the way of my life.

Depression is a part of my Asperger's and is often triggered by the frustration of wanting to get my life together and relate better to people around me.

Anxiety is also part and parcel of having Asperger's. For some reason, we feel things more intensely. I remember having my first panic or anxiety attack while in Kalgoorlie at the tender age of eight. It was a really hot day at a sports carnival. I started hyperventilating, breathing really fast, and getting very dizzy in the process. I was so scared because I didn't understand what was going on with me and I really thought that I was going to die. I remember lying on the ground with one or two teachers looking at me and a few students gathered around. I didn't understand what was happening and I felt really hot. I could have had a touch of heatstroke, perhaps. It was really embarrassing for me having other people seeing me in the state I was in. I think they told my parents about what happened and they made sure I rested quietly that night. That was my first anxiety attack and many have followed during my life.

Being Taken Advantage Of

Unfortunately, Aspies often are naive and too trusting of people and end up in situations where they are used, abused and taken advantage of. As I've mentioned, when I was a kid I was very friendly and would hug and touch strangers. When I was three years old, a teenage guy my family was looking after exposed himself to me in his bedroom. I remember seeing his penis really close up with white stuff on the tip of it. One of my parents came in and found us. 'Bruiser' was sent away the next day but I was pretty freaked out after that experience and I think it shaped my behaviour as a kid in quite a few different ways.

The following is part of a piece I wrote almost 20 years ago. I actually wrote it as an article to submit to a women's or teen magazine to try to help other people. I was a teenager when I wrote this piece. Of course, you don't have to have Asperger's to be the victim of sexual abuse, but the problems with communicating and not understanding people makes it all the more likely that Aspies will end up in bad situations.

It Couldn't Happen To Me! October, 1990

There are those out there who have been hurt by sexual abuse. I'm writing this to those who have been hurt, and also the lucky ones who haven't, to let you know what it feels like. It is a common thing in Australia but it is also a well-known secret. You know of it through gossip and think it's not going to happen to you, that is until it does. It can happen to anyone. It doesn't have to be serious to leave emotional scars on you. Rape is the most serious one, but fortunately mine wasn't that serious. This is my story:

AGE: 13 years

PLACE: A church camp

FRIDAY: Another church camp with heaps of exciting things to do and see. Mum and dad aren't here so it's my very first camp without them, ever. Tonight we had a sing-a-long and it was excellent seeing all my old friends again after one whole year. I'm really looking forward to all the fun times of this weekend.

SUNDAY: Last night something happened to me that I couldn't understand. I cannot describe this strange feeling which comes from the pit of my stomach. It happened during the concert and no-one saw. I was abused by this guy, a member of one of the churches. I think he's 10–15 years older than me. Some of us were walking down to the river and, as we started walking across the oval, his hand started going down my shirt slowly and then I got scared. When we got there we all sat down on the bench and started talking.

Then suddenly he sent them away for something and I was left with him. He then started talking to me about the river and the night but all the while his hand kept touching me. It seemed evil and threatening to me. Finally, after what seemed like hours the boys got back and the concert had finished also. So that was a big relief.

MONDAY: Today he abused me again and I'm feeling really confused. I think somehow I asked for more but I don't know how. Today I was down on the oval just playing around and he called me into his room because he said he wanted to speak to me. I came hesitantly and he tried to make me feel comfortable by smiling at me. I stayed at the door ready to move if he came towards me. He started talking to me about the weekend and how he enjoyed it.

I asked him why he touched me and he didn't answer but instead told me not to ever tell anyone about it. Then came the lure, he invited me into his room and said I could try to play his guitar. I accepted the sugar-coated offer. Maybe he wouldn't do it again I thought innocently. He gave me the guitar to play around with and he continued packing his things.

A few minutes passed and then he came over to me, took away my flimsy source of security (the guitar) and started kissing me and touching me up my shirt. At that moment I froze completely and pretended it wasn't happening to me again. About10 minutes later he suddenly stopped, quickly gave me back the guitar and he told me to play it. He went and pretended to pack. A moment later his roommate arrived and asked pleasantly how we were. I looked up and smiled weakly and said I was fine. They started talking to each other and I quickly made my escape.

I know what it feels like and if it happens to you, tell someone you trust or tell one of your teachers at school or your parents especially. The best way to do it is to tell them right away. I hope I have helped you in some way, shape or form. Just remember that anyone can abuse you but never, never think it couldn't happen to you, because it just might.

Sexual Abuse

Have you ever been hurt?
Have you ever been abused?
Have you ever been lonely?
I know what it feels like
The hurt cuts deep like a knife
The abuse stays in the pit of the stomach
The loneliness doesn't go away
I know what it feels like

How Asperger's Has Affected Me

A painful fact of life
Nearly drowning sometimes
Your bitter years later
I know what it feels like
Too scared to get close to someone
Trust is gone and severed
Men are killers of the soul
I know what it feels like
They devour it and ask for more
Many people go through it
Your revenge is being strong
I know what it feels like
A secret that is painful
But you are not alone
There are millions out there
I know what it feels like
A crime for being a woman
An object of fantasy and lust
With no feelings or emotions
I know what it feels like
You feel cheap and dirty
And you blame yourself
But it's not your fault
I know what it feels like
We are a team
We stick together
Believe me ...
I know what it feels like.

© Megan Hammond,1990

I had not read this in many years and had a couple of sleepless nights over it when I retyped it. It seems like half a lifetime ago, when I was so young and innocent. Even today I have really mixed feelings about it. I found it more confusing than most to deal with something like this, I think, but writing this, I felt that I could express my feelings better.

When I was 16 years old I had to deal with the Wolfie scenarios and they really put a spanner in the works for me with regard to trusting people. It was a very lonely time, when I felt completely isolated from everyone around me.

In my 20s, just before I was diagnosed with Asperger's, I was taken advantage of by a man from church who was engaged. He saw how vulnerable I was, 'groomed' me and then went in for the kill so to speak. He told me to tell no-one because they wouldn't understand … the classic line people like that say. About six months later I told a trusted friend who said I should tell the fiancée and the associate pastor. Anyway, it all came out into the open and I lost quite a few friends because of it. No-one believed me and maybe thought I was crazy.

So even as an adult the wool still gets pulled over my eyes. As an older person I still do not know or understand why these things happened to me. I can't get inside anybody's head to really know what someone is thinking. All I know is that there are some people out there who see weakness and vulnerability in someone and decide to 'groom' them for their own means. It can be about power, sex or control or a combination of all of these. It's very complicated.

I have forgiven but not forgotten, and I am stronger for it. Sometimes I wonder if these guys abused other kids in their lifetimes. Have they or will they ever get caught?

Now I am the type of person who will stand up and say something about these issues instead of leaving them hidden, buried underneath shame and much guilt. I know that there are others out there like me who have been through similar experiences. I have discovered my voice now and I will speak out about issues I've been silent about for many years.

~

Perhaps one of the biggest problems for people with Asperger's is relationships and how to relate to others appropriately. I am told that most people simply 'know' intuitively what the correct thing to do is in various situations, particularly as they grow up. For some reason, Aspies just don't know how to act and actually have to think and remember each time what is the right thing to do in each situation.

It gets even trickier when we fall in love—everybody's brain gets a bit scrambled then. Just think how hard it is for me!

9

Finding—And Losing—Love

For a long time I wondered why relationships were such a mystery to me, but after my diagnosis with Asperger's the jigsaw pieces began to fit together. One of the main traits of Asperger's is not knowing how to communicate effectively and appropriately with others. Especially with people close to you.

In my life I have had only four serious relationships. Each of these has affected me in different ways.

Alex, Brookvale, 1991

In 1990, at 18 years of age, I began attending Christian City Church in Brookvale, a church that was attended mainly by young people. One evening, on Sunday, 5 May 1991, a very ordinary night with crowds of people everywhere, I was talking to a friend of mine. Michael said that he would like to introduce me to a friend of his who had happened to come along that night. I was still busy talking to someone else and turned to be introduced to this new guy.

To our surprise we looked at each other and remembered at the same time we were long lost childhood friends! He said, 'Megan! ... Megan Hammond?'

I said, virtually at the same time, 'Alex! ... Alex, is that YOU?'

With huge grins on our faces we fell into a big hug that seemed to last for minutes. We kept talking, ignoring everyone around us. It was like we were in our own little world catching up on the many years. We couldn't believe we were meeting each other again. The next morning I discovered a letter on the doorstep. He had cycled several kilometres to our home the night before and left it there as a surprise.

From that night we were virtually inseparable for almost the next three years. That was the longest relationship that I've ever had. Alex and I were totally mad about each other, which everyone saw. We did so much together and through him I learned many different things— bike riding, skiing, improving my fitness, determination, romance—I trusted him totally and thought he'd be the only man in my life no matter what.

He had a tall, strong, muscular figure, and stood 1.88 metres (6 foot 2 inches) tall, definitely something every woman would love. He was born in Australia but his half-Dutch, half-Maltese heritage really shone out. With his Roman nose and deep brown eyes he looked to me like a Greek god.

Every time I was around him I would melt and sometimes he would also. Sometimes we'd just look into each other's eyes with tears in them and say 'I love you!' to each other. We'd both be there with tears running down our faces and these stupid big goofy smiles, then end up in a huge, tight bear hug.

Those hugs I thought would never end in a million years. We felt so safe in each other's embrace where no-one could ever touch us. The world was ours for us to conquer and explore and nothing could stop us, not even our parents.

A few months into the relationship we secretly got engaged but I didn't get a ring. He was still in high school finishing his HSC so we were both quite strapped for cash. His parents must have been worried whether he was going to actually pass his HSC or not.

The times I had with Alex were both beautiful yet turbulent. We were very much in love with each other. He was my one true love and he changed my life forever. As most couples do, we had our ups and downs and were way too young for the relationship to succeed properly. Although I had learned so much in many different ways, during my time with Alex I still had some demons raging away in me.

'Hey, I don't think we're working out, but I still love you!' Alex's voice rattled around his small Peugeot car.

'I know, Alex. Everything seems so different in a lot of ways from when we started out.'

The day was rainy and grey, just like our moods. We were at the top of Dee Why headland overlooking the water with seagulls buzzing around the car like flies. We found ourselves in our familiar embrace but with sad tears in our eyes.

'You know that we've given it our best shot don't you?' he asked tenderly, looking down at me.

'Yes I know we have. I was sure we were going to get married one day. I thought we were going to be together forever as we promised.'

But the fairytale was over and the cracks were showing everywhere. It was time to say farewell to a young man who had meant so much to me. Eventually, in February 1994, we broke up.

During those years that we were together I totally blossomed as a woman and my life had a dramatic turnaround. Alex was the best thing that had ever happened to me. We both helped each other and learned about love through each other in a lot of different ways. He was like my knight in shining armour—not rescuing me, just sharing himself with me during those years. I will always remember him with the fondest of memories.

And wherever he is I wish him the best happiness that life has to offer him!

~

Despite my relationship with Alex, since my mid-teens I had felt an attraction to other women. I found myself still struggling with this.

Later in 1994 I was on a quest to find out who I really was and to try to align the two forces—my attraction to women and also being

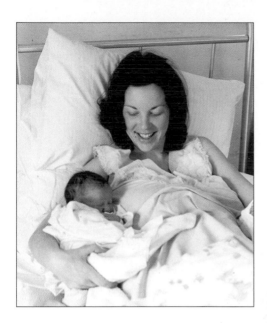

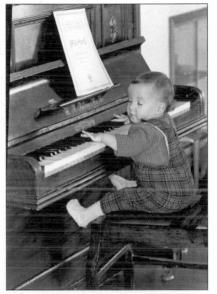

Above: I make my debut with mum, Sally.
Right: I always liked music, here I am
showing a particular fondness for
Brahms.
Below: I was fascinated by the contents
of the kitchen cupboards and obviously
surprised to see Dad inside the cupboard
waiting for me to open the door.

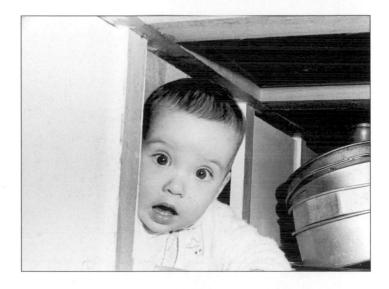

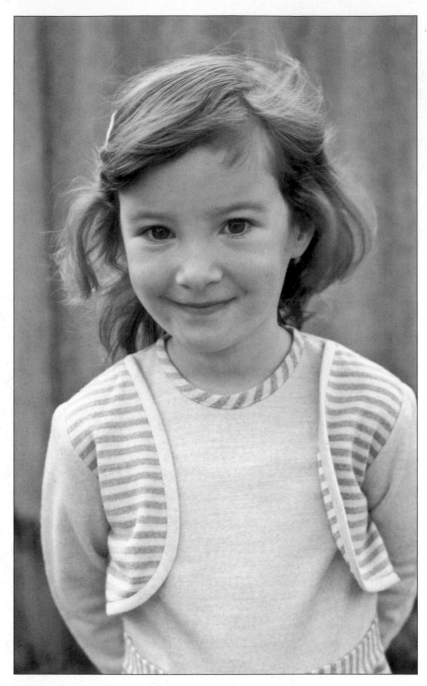

Dressed up for church in Geraldton, Western Australia in 1977. I would rather have been wearing jeans.

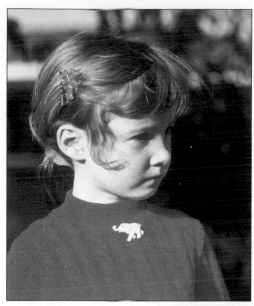

Left: People saw me as a quiet little girl—1975 with Mum's elephant brooch (Below) My first overseas trip, in Switzerland, 1976. My brother Cam and I had just seen snow for the first time.

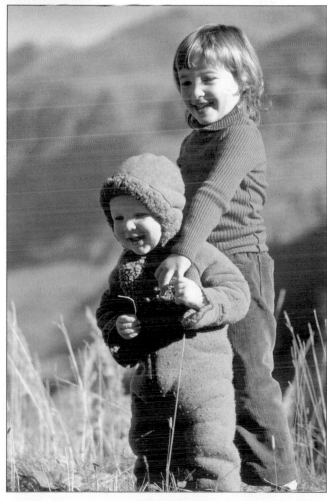

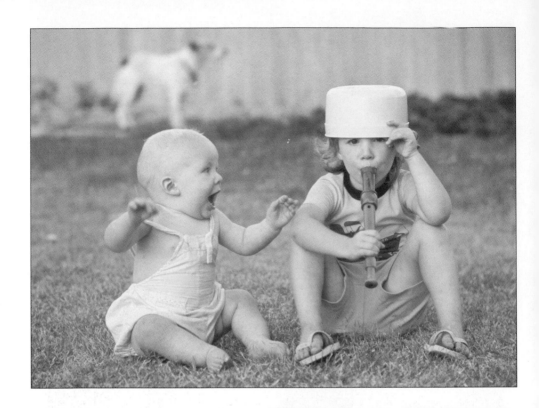

Above: Cameron thought I was very funny. Geraldton, Western Australia, 1976.
(Right) The two of us when we moved to Sydney, 1982.
(Below) In 1996 I took a visit to Western Australia, to catch up with old friends.

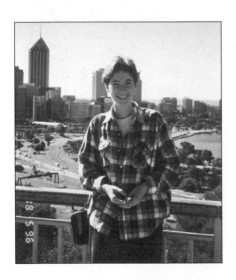

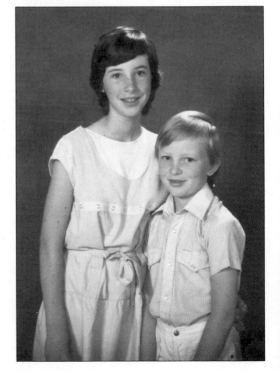

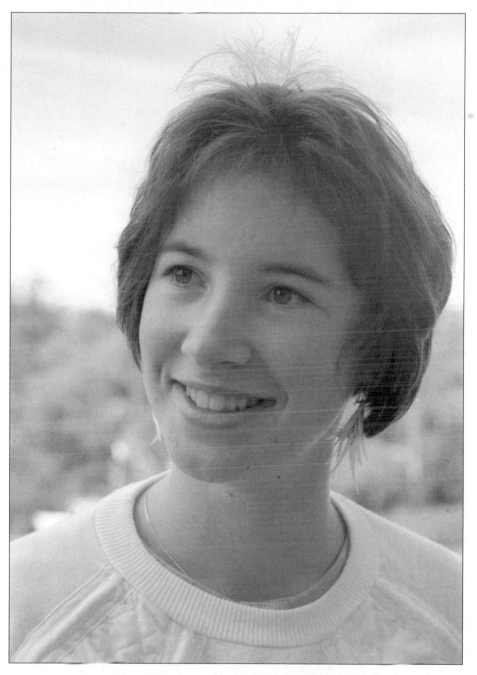

Sweet 16 (I hardly think so) in Brookvale, New South Wales. Turbulent years.

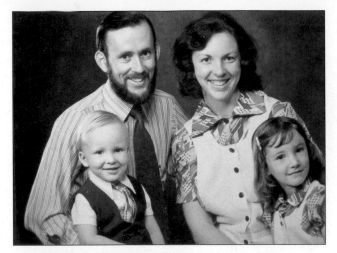

Family photos. Geraldton, Western Australia, 1977.

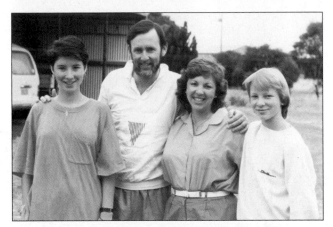

A visit to Esperance, Western Australia, in 1988.

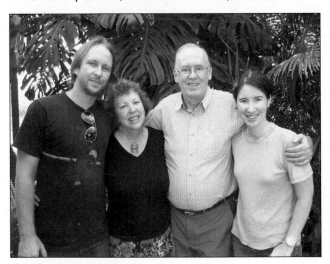

Christmas Day, 2008.

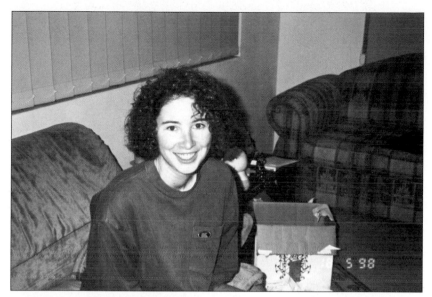

In 1998 I moved into my unit. At last I had a place I could call my own.

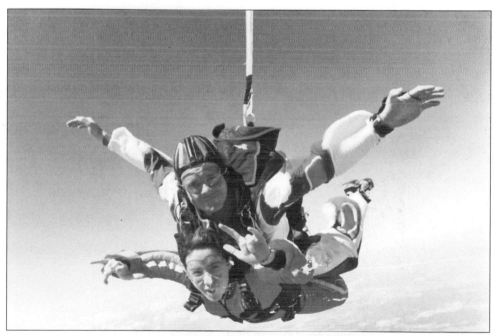

A leap into the unknown. My first skydive near Cessnock in 2004.

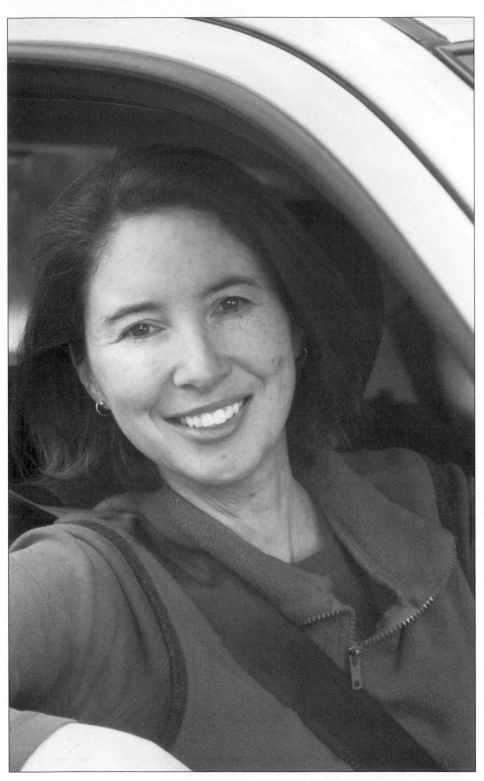

Behind the wheel of my car in 2009. I am in control, I am free and this is one place where I feel no different to anybody else.

a Christian—that were pulling me apart inside. I needed to put them to rest even though they seemed to be polar opposites in a lot of different ways.

I started going to a young lesbian support group without my parents or friends really knowing. Something was pulling me towards those people who had similar feelings to me and which I found comforting. I had no idea of the violence that would befall me the following year.

Suzie, 1995

I couldn't believe my eyes and what I was seeing. Suzie pulled the phone out of my hand and threw it hard against the wall.

'Oh my crumbs! What have I done?' I asked in a shocked stilted manner.

'You! You! I'm angry…!' Her voice trailed off with her eyes ablaze with fiery fury.

She sat down on the lounge drinking her longneck of VB beer, preparing another cone for herself. I stood there shaking as an icy atmosphere came over the room.

'What should I do? What am I going to do here?' I quietly said in my mind. Would she read my thoughts through the silence of the room?

I didn't want another outburst of anger so I sat on the other end of the lounge and lit up my cigarette quietly so as not to annoy her. I looked sideways at her, all hunched over and tense like stone, concentrating on getting the cone ready for herself. Slowly she put the bong up to her mouth, breathing in hard and holding it in for a while. Breathing out finally, the smoke filled the air and her face looked even harder, more jaded, lost.

She didn't say a thing and instantly started preparing another cone for herself, which didn't surprise me. After my cigarette I walked over to the phone by the wall to look at it. It had one or two cracks in it and no cord because Suzie was still holding onto it.

'Don't worry, I'll try to fix the phone later. I'm used to this … Looks like there's no more phone calls for you for the rest of the night! Now your parents can't interfere with our lives!'

I turned around and looked at her, stunned, unable to say anything. She gave me a sarcastic smile and had another gulp of the beer she was clutching.

This is going to be another long night, I thought sadly. I hope I get through it without her getting any angrier. In my 22 years no-one had ever treated me this way.

~

A few weeks later I was off in my own little world, walking behind Suzie to our unit one night. Next thing I hear: Crash! Thud, tinkle, tinkle!

Bloody hell! What's happened now? I thought.

Coming closer to Suzie I noticed that one of the unit's outside doors was broken. Suzie was glaring at me with bloodshot stoned eyes. 'Look what you've made me do, you dirty slut!' she sneered.

'What? What, I wasn't even near the door!' I stammered.

'If it wasn't for you I wouldn't be drinking all the time and angry! You're the cause of all this! ...,' she continued on with her tirade.

Her barrage of insults continued to pierce my heart like arrows. We finally got upstairs to our unit and she poured a drink of spirits for us both. She sat on the floor motioning me to sit down also. I was hesitant but sat cross-legged facing her. She sucked back a cone that she had prepared for herself.

'Let's talk about things and be honest!' Her slurred words came out, hitting me full-on.

'Now honestly! Have you ever thought about being with anyone else?' she asked me.

'No I don't think I have,' came my honest answer.

Next thing I knew I felt a hard, heavy blow against my face. She'd hit me. The sudden sting shocked me.

'You're lying, you fucking slut! I know you are, you dirty cunt!' Her voice came pounding across to me.

Another stinging hit landed on the other side of my face. She then sneered again saying … 'I'm going to keep hitting you until the truth comes out! Even if it takes all night, you bitch!'

I just sat there stunned, unable to comprehend what was going on.

'What about your curry-munching, stinking, ugly friend? And that woman at your work, you bitch!' she continued on.

Interrupting her I managed to say, 'No I haven't! I've always been faithful to you! I wouldn't even think about it. Have you thought of being with anyone else?'

The air was deadly silent for one second, then the screaming banshee was released and I felt a few more hard hits around my face that brought tears to my eyes instantly.

Her voice rose. 'No way, you fucking piece of spoilt rubbish! Who do you think you are, you stupid bitch! You've got no idea, you slut! You're so stupid!'

By this time I was feeling confused and defeated. Tears were clearly staining my face now. I felt so lost and alone in the world that I couldn't help but cry. It was like Suzie the cat was playing with me, the mouse, in a cruel, sadistic game where I'd always be the loser no matter which way I turned.

She had her heavy paw on me and I was unable to move, however hard I tried. I began to doubt everything about my life and myself when I was with her. It was almost like I was her puppet and she was pulling the strings. I was a totally different person who I hardly recognised anymore.

When I went to bed that night, I couldn't rest properly because of all the things going around in my mind. Trying to deal with an angry and violent girlfriend was all new and confusing. I was not used to dealing with people like that. It was like I was dying on the inside, but on the outside I was still living and breathing, trying to put up a front.

At work the next day I must have looked a sight with little red marks and bruises on my face along with a fat lip and bruised ears. Trying to concentrate on the job of putting components into circuit boards and soldering them up correctly was so hard when I was tired beyond belief. The abuse had been escalating for a couple of months. Sometimes

I'd burn my hands or fingers accidentally because of lapses in my concentration. Then I'd go home where the abuse would sometimes start all over again or I'd be walking on eggshells very carefully so that I didn't upset her.

I don't know how I managed to get through those days of pure hell.

~

The year 1995 was a huge year for me in a lot of different ways. It left a wound on my soul that I am still living with today. If I could turn back time I would in an instant. I would change everything and make it right again. Yet in life you can't do that.

Suzie and I met at a pub early one March morning. We were sitting beside each other on the stairs having a cigarette. Somehow we got talking and she seemed to be sad—sad and stoned. I knew little about pot at that point in time.

I wasn't attracted to her, simply making polite conversation. She had a rough appearance.

Next thing, the bar staff yelled out, 'Last drinks. Bar is now closed! Come on. Time to go, guys!'

As we got up from where we were sitting I noticed she was quite a bit shorter than me, but she had an air of toughness about her.

We exchanged phone numbers and I drove back home to Brookvale. I mentioned something about meeting Suzie to my parents. We called each other over the next few days and met up a few more times. Always in the back of my mind were my parents' words: 'Megan, we're worried that this woman's not that good for you.' Their faces were ghostly white shadows in my mind's eye.

In mid-March Suzie asked me to be her girlfriend and I said 'Yes!' I was like a red sore thumb standing out in a crowd waiting to be hammered.

At this time she was staying in a block of flats that had a bad reputation for violence, alcohol and drugs. It was a whole new world to me and

I slid further down into the gaping abyss that was Suzie's world. She became my siren, the voice I listened to above any others in my life.

I moved in with her and we created our own little world of listening to music, smoking cigarettes, drinking a lot and smoking pot. We were inseparable. I didn't particularly want to go home to my parents because I felt uncomfortable about my new life.

My poor parents were freaking out. Our phone conversations were very uncomfortable and they were asking me things like, 'Are you a lesbian now?' and 'What are you doing?' and other questions which I couldn't answer properly.

They wanted me home, tucked up in my own little bed, safe and sound away from all this bad stuff.

~

After months of abuse and escalating anger and violence, it had to happen.

'I'm breaking up with you because we're not working out!' Suzie's voice on the phone was cold. I was at work at the time and as soon as I heard that I could've dropped to the floor!

'Um ... arr ... but, wait!' My stumbling reply burbled out through my mouth, the receiver shaking in my hand.

As soon as work finished I drove madly to Glebe, where we were now living. Desperation gripped me in its deadly claw as I parked the car. Our unit was empty. I cracked completely. My mind was blank and next thing I knew I found myself throwing something against the wall. Then something else was thrown ... it was like watching a movie of a stranger going crazy. Not me. It was like I couldn't control myself or I was possessed by some evil spirit. A huge volcano of feeling exploded inside me, overpowering me. I continued on until the flat was a mess, then left to drive and sort out my feelings.

We were together for almost two years, counting all the break-ups and getting together again. It turned into a devilish cycle of some happy times, where hope blossomed, then cruelty followed by another angry break-up, a reunion, then torturous hope. To be bashed, abused, even raped by another woman—your own sex—is a truly harrowing and traumatising experience. You are being hurt and betrayed by one of your sisterhood.

The violence I experienced at Suzie's hands was so demeaning that the after-effects of it still nearly kill me with the shame, and with great sadness. For many years afterwards I suffered immense devastation, feeling completely isolated from everybody.

Even though I have learned greatly from these experiences and have been able to forgive, that doesn't mean that I'm unaffected by them. But the way I see it, another day lived is another day of getting stronger and understanding more about life.

I have been forever changed by those experiences. I endured untold pain—physical, spiritual and psychological—and I'm a wiser person now so I can be there for other people if they ever need me.

After something like that there is no kind of 'normal' anymore.

Dave, Brookvale, 1997

The relationship with Suzie took a really bad turn and late in 1996 I ended up in a clinic to help deal with the effects of the abuse I had been subjected to. It was here that I met Dave. He had been suffering from depression.

We both had different hassles going on and became firm friends, something we both needed at the time. He was understanding and caring and we could relate to each other.

Later on that year, at a cafe in Glebe, we met again at an ex-patients' reunion. After that we stayed in regular contact and started seeing movies together. It wasn't until early in 1997 that we were in the movies and held hands very shyly. We realised that the feeling was mutual and started to go out as a couple, taking it really slowly together. Both of us had been through some pretty rough times and didn't want to run full-on into a relationship that would end in tears, yet again.

Dave was a few years younger than me but he was such a gentle sweet guy and I really connected with him. I loved him in my own way and we were together on and off until 1999, then remained extremely good friends after that. At the time that we were going out I was determined to do the right thing by God and myself. I was going to church and wasn't planning to have sex until marriage no matter who wanted it. I was saving myself for someone who was worth it after the abusive relationship with Suzie.

Dave and I never did have sex but I was tempted at the time a lot. I never acted on those feelings, though, which was maybe good in the long run because it made it easier for us to be friends afterwards.

He was a very special young man I cared deeply about and always will. He was a true, gentle-natured spirit who gave me back some confidence in men in general. Dave didn't care that my last relationship was with an abusive woman, he just wanted me and us as a couple to be happy. Finally we let each other go. Last I heard was he was engaged and soon to be married.

My best relationship, 2006

In the last half of 2005 I enrolled in a writing course. In 2006 we were all given the option of doing an advanced course that was aimed at giving us the basics of writing a book. Nearly all of us—eight students, each with different interests—decided to keep going with it, and a few new faces turned up, including someone who was closer to my age.

I remember thinking to myself, 'Good! They're mostly older women and I'm NOT going to be attracted to any of them! It's just going to be a healing time of friendships for me.'

Ruth did notice me, however, and was attracted to me as a person. The next few months flew by and we became really good friends. I took her out to lunch for her birthday after our writing group had finished that day and her friendly smile showed her appreciation. During the holidays we met up a few times. She was a single mother, which I understood, and didn't mind about at all.

Meeting her at this time was very interesting as neither of us expected to meet or become involved with anyone; and anyway, we were just good friends.

The turning point came in October when we had lunch in Avalon and spent the afternoon together talking and sharing. I realised that I was starting to become really attracted to her—more than just a friend. This was frustrating for me, because as far as I knew she was straight and had never been with women before. So I decided not to tell her about my growing feelings in case she freaked out over it.

We still talked on the phone a lot and when the course resumed after the holidays we again had our usual lunches and sharing time afterwards on Wednesday afternoons.

Later that month most of the women, including us, went away for a writing weekend. It was a really big weekend of writing and also sharing and I felt myself becoming even more attracted to her. I wanted to give her great big hugs and hold her hands, but there was no way in the world that was possible.

On the Saturday night I couldn't sleep much so I wrote out my feelings of how I was attracted to someone straight. I so wanted to tell her how I felt during that weekend, but I didn't.

A short time afterwards we were having lunch on a really windy, cold day after writing. I gave her my jacket to wear because she was quite cold. Looking over the bay there on the harbour I did eventually tell her that I was attracted to a straight woman but I didn't have the guts to tell her that it was her. We parted ways with our normal big goodbye hugs and that was it. I was determined to try to forget about her so I could move on.

That night I got a phone call from her wanting to ask me a few questions. After the initial conversation she asked, 'Um, Megan … am I the straight woman that you're attracted to?'

'Um, okay. Why do you want to know that?' I responded.

She continued, 'I'm just getting a feeling that it could be me that you like.'

We talked for a bit and I was so nervous about it.

Then I asked, 'Why, are you attracted to me or something?'

Her answer came back, 'Yes, Megan, I do like you a lot and yes, I am attracted to you too!'

On my end of the phone I couldn't believe my ears and I had this huge goofy grin on my face. I told her, 'Yes, I like you a lot too. Yes, you are the straight woman who I've liked as well!'

The barriers came down as we realised that we did have a mutual attraction for one another and both felt like schoolgirls again talking to each other on the phone. We had to see each other really soon after that and made plans for me to go over to her house on the Sunday afternoon.

Driving over there that afternoon I was so nervous and was running a bit late. When I arrived at the house she saw my car stop outside and came to meet me, giving me a big, tight hug. We went into her house where we talked a lot about different things and also us. She had cooked a special dinner and we washed it down with numerous glasses of water and cups of tea.

I was on a massive natural high, but within the space of a month she broke it off with me because she was not used to being in a steady relationship and was battling health issues.

This began a yoyo series of break-ups and getting back together over the next two years. I felt confused. After finding someone again who had melted my icy barriers, suddenly I was alone again.

Leaving me to pick up the pieces all over again has been sad and very hard for me. She was the best girlfriend that I've ever had and she genuinely cared for and loved me. The times we had were very special. Each day I try to remember that life does go on and that there is a future ahead for me here!

~

While these stories of my relationships may seem very personal, they need to be told. Like anyone else I long to be loved and cared for and have someone of my own to love too, but so often I misread the cues, or else others simply don't understand me. Trying to comprehend or understand people is a hard task for anyone. Having Asperger's syndrome makes it even harder—it's like marching to the beat of your own drum. Not quite in synch with everybody else, we are always three steps or so behind understanding the true actions or intentions of people around us. I sometimes find it extremely hard to relate to friends and family in a mature way.

10

Falling Through The Cracks
And Finding My Feet

For so long no-one, including the doctors, has known where to put me or what label to assign me so they can put me in a nice little pigeonhole.

I kept falling through small cracks in different situations. As the years passed it felt that the cracks had turned into deep canyons and as if one wrong step could be my last. If I fell I would be lost, confused or trying to climb out of that hole for a very long time indeed. I had to make my own path and find my own feet in the world, which I feel I've done in a sense.

There are a few areas where I've fallen through the cracks: support services, education and employment, society in general, and religion, but I have come to deal with life in my own way. Even though I've given up a few times I always found the strength to go on with my family's, friends' and God's help.

Adults with Asperger's, like me, fall through the cracks in the health system too. Because the condition is neither a physical nor a mental disability, there is currently not a big enough bucket of money assigned to assisting us Aspies.

Support Services

As I have mentioned, when I was a kid my parents took me to many doctors, speech therapists, occupational therapists and specialists to try to find out what was wrong with me. One GP in the 1980s even misdiagnosed me with OCD (Obsessive Compulsive Disorder), going as far as saying that I would end up living in an institution for the rest of my life. Well, I guess I proved him wrong, because I've got my own place, which is a haven for me.

Although I managed to find jobs and joined up with the CES (Commonwealth Employment Service) and Social Security when I couldn't find any work, both those services had no idea how to really serve or support me because they couldn't work me out. I was just another long-term unemployed citizen who they had to get off their books and out to a job for the efficiency of their system.

One time I was sent on a course that was for really disabled people because I wasn't diagnosed at the time with Asperger's. I found it really off-putting.

There are clinics, which I attended for my emotional problems including major depression and getting over my abusive ex, and for help trying to get other issues sorted out. However, the major difficulty with these places was that I found myself mixing with mentally ill people and others with alcohol and substance-abuse problems. I began to think I might have those problems too, and I also picked up anti-social behaviours and made some friends there who ultimately were not good for me.

So for many years I was passed over and nearly forgotten until the significant year when I was finally diagnosed.

The goal then was to put me in touch with services that would help me because I was still in no fit state to work or try to find a job of any sort. After a lifetime of knock-backs, being passed about and puzzled over, I was emotionally down the drain, lost somewhere there, stuck and unable to move. My life had to be slowly unravelled with care on all the different levels where things had happened.

Later on in that year, 1998, after my diagnosis, I was put on the Disability Support Pension to help out with my financial problems and in 1999 I was referred to the CRS (Commonwealth Rehabilitation Service), which did help to a degree.

In 2000 I got about two months' work experience at a video store through a support officer from the CRS. I felt like I was succeeding in some way and slowly getting my life back together. In 2001 they helped me get some voluntary work with Community Aid Abroad and also in bringing my résumé more up to date, which needed to be done. It was around that time when the worker who was looking after me at CRS left, and it was decided that they couldn't really help me anymore.

My mum also contacted the Autism Society. They told us that they didn't have any support for adults with Asperger's, but they had plenty of services for kids. They did tell her about the Asperger's Social Group, which ran every two weeks, for young adults and adults with Asperger's. There was a calendar of different activities and they sent her a contact number to call the organisers. Over the next half year mum was going to try for us to have a cup of coffee and talk with one of the organisers. But mum was really busy with work and travelling and the organisers were on the other side of the city, so we never got around to it. She gave me the calendar and I contacted the organisers, feeling so nervous and scared that it wasn't funny.

The lady in charge invited me to a movie night at the cinemas in Burwood so I went, not knowing what to expect. I had never met another adult with Asperger's before and here's me in my 30s! I remember thinking, what are they going to look like? How bad are they going to be? How many people will there be? What's the age range going to be like? Are there going to be many other women? (The reason for that question is because Asperger's is more common in males.) Most importantly, are they going to be friendly? These and a load of other questions were going through my head as I was driving there.

When I arrived at Burwood I quickly had a cigarette to help calm my nerves and then I walked in and managed to find one of the group leaders. She in turn introduced me to about 12 to 15 other people. One or two of them were actually parents of people there. I was glad to see that there were one or two other women and felt a bit more comfortable.

We all went and saw the various movies the group had chosen and then met up later in the foyer for a quick talk before leaving. I arrived home with a deep sense of relief and satisfaction that I did finally make it to one of the outings after so long, and met other people with the same condition as me. I felt that I was no longer alone—on quite a few different levels of the word—for the first time in my life.

~

Around 2004 my mum heard that the Autism Society was going to offer some type of support as well as a skills course for adults with Asperger's syndrome, which was exactly what I needed to help get me started back in the workforce. However, soon after this there were a lot of staff changes at the society as well as lack of government funding, I think, so they kept putting the date for beginning the new service further off, saying the beginning of the next year, and so on. Eventually they had to call it off for whatever reasons, which was hugely disappointing for me.

In late 2008 when I was doing some research on the internet I found that ASPECT, which was originally known as the Autism Society, was going to organise Aspect Community Participation Services and a post-school options course in 2009. It seemed to be designed for adults with Asperger's syndrome or autism spectrum disorders; teaching, supporting and helping them learn a huge range of skills, and other activities.

As soon as I saw that web link I decided to email the people in charge expressing my interest. The holy grail of services had just plonked down in my lap and I was going to grab it with both hands. During the next few days I let a lot of my friends know, including the ladies in the writing group. Checking my emails a week later I found that it was a totally different story. The lady who was supposedly in charge replied to me in her email saying she was not involved in the Asperger's program and referred me to her boss.

A couple of days later he replied to me saying that while there was a social group, 'Aspect currently does not provide any specific service to adults with Asperger's.' He added that the society was trying to get a program funded.

I became even more confused and frustrated and decided to send them a combined email stating my feelings. I also included the web link to the page pointing out exactly where on their site I had found this information. There were also a few questions that I wanted to know the answers to, which hopefully they knew.

Another few days passed and then the reply came from the director saying, '…unfortunately Asperger's is not funded as other disability categories are. Because there is no IQ issue then people with Asperger's are not eligible for DADHC funding…we are trying to get greater recognition for this group of people and hopefully a funded program'.

Fallen through the cracks again!

Society

I'm just a little bit different from everyone else around me in this society. All my life I have been trying to fit in as best I can. I'm not a fringe dweller, but I have attracted quite a few dodgy people in my life who haven't had my best interests at heart. Sometimes I've fallen in with the wrong crowd and it has taken me ages to get myself out. They've included people with mental illnesses, a church group, people who drank a lot as well as used drugs, people who used me and took advantage of me for various reasons (both straight and homosexual people), and a few churchgoers as well.

Here I've mentioned people from vastly different sections of society, so in truth I have met a very wide variety of people throughout my life. In this way I think that I could be quite different to most people because I may have seen things that others around me have never seen before. For quite a while I was living in the extreme parallel universes of church on the one hand and a drinking, partying and mostly homosexual crowd on the other. But I was still me throughout those periods and was honest with both sets of friends about what I was doing with the other group.

For example, sometimes on a Saturday night I'd hang around a drinking crowd and then go to church on the Sunday evening, sometimes in the morning if I wasn't too tired. I also still had my own set of personal guidelines and morals that I would stand by, but I've tried new things sometimes to see what they were like.

Mum told me something important a long time ago: 'Megs, you don't have to be an open book to everyone. Nobody really needs to know your business if you don't want them to. You don't have to tell people everything about yourself!'

I took that on board and decided to be more private and discreet about some things until I could trust certain people around me. Even then sometimes when I told someone about my varied life they would be really surprised. Some people couldn't understand how I could be involved in such conflicting activities (going to church on Sundays and then on weekends clubbing and drinking at pubs—occasionally staying out all night), but I needed the variety, the spice in my life, to keep it interesting. That's just me: a varied, interesting person who does not easily conform to society's standards.

Over the years a lot of people around me have tried to put different labels on me. Some of them have been accurate but many others haven't. Even a couple of professionals have disagreed with my discomfort about being stereotyped. One such label is in regard to my sexuality, which is really no-one else's business. When people have asked me whether I'm straight or a lesbian, my standard answer is, 'I'm not gay, bisexual, lesbian, transgender or whatever ... I am just me—and that's it!'

Nowadays I don't tell people that type of thing unless I know them quite well. I don't like advertising different parts about myself because to me they are really personal and private. I don't say anything unless I ultimately have to. But I can also still definitely stand up for myself on certain issues. Even so, I've been learning to try to be more easygoing, and to hear other people out with an open mind, which I feel is also important.

Despite at times feeling very alone, sometimes on my way down I've noticed that other people fall through the cracks of society as well: the elderly and even more disabled people, some with even rarer conditions than mine. I guess we all have our own cross to bear in this life. Yes I do admit that sometimes I forget that there are people worse off than me, but I guess that's an average flaw that we all have as human beings in this world.

Sure I've fallen in with the wrong people sometimes and I don't fit neatly into society's labels. But I have made my own way with the help of my family, friends and also people from church who have stuck by me. I've found my feet and am leading my own individual way of life, which does have its ups and downs. I'm not perfect and have got heaps still to learn but I have my dignity and sense of self, which is really important. I have achieved a lot in the last few years and appreciate things more as well.

~

There is one item that has been in the news over the past year or so which has been very sad for me. This was the fatal stabbing and subsequent death of a young man who had Asperger's syndrome. I never met Gerard Fleming but he was well known in his community. Gerard was 35 years of age when he died on 16 June 2007. The event took place at the Narrabeen Tramshed toilets late one cold winter's night. There was also an electrical storm happening that night when a neighbour heard banging and kicking in the toilets. Little did she know what was really happening there. Gerard was later found on the footpath near a bus stop where he'd actually dragged himself after the attack. Somebody notified the ambulance and it was then he told the ambulance officers who it was that had attacked him in the toilets.

Gerard was also a Christian and was well known to the local shopkeepers of that area. To those who knew him or met him he was friendly, really good-natured, gentle and childlike. He had a high intelligence but some people could take him the wrong way. A lot of people turned up for his funeral, which showed how much the stabbing had affected the community.

Over the following months of investigation the Tramshed toilets were labelled by the media as being a 'gay beat'. The police did track down the teenager who killed Gerard Fleming and he was taken into custody. He was charged with Gerard's death, then the case was taken to court. It was said that the incident between them both happened because of a failure to communicate. During the court case the charge of murder was reduced to manslaughter. The teenager has been sent to jail for this crime.

For me this stabbing death of another young person like myself with Asperger's, which is often called a mild form of autism (or high-functioning autism), is very telling. Although he had certain vulnerabilities and problems with communication and relating to people, Gerard still had a good heart. No-one will probably ever know exactly what happened in those last hours of his life but his story has really touched me.

My guess is that he experienced the same type of struggles as me with different pressures and society. I am sorry that he had to die to get Asperger's syndrome in the media. Gerard Fleming was a unique young man and he will always be in the memories of his family, friends, those who knew him and also me. I hope that through his death we can learn more as a community, and a society as a whole.

Religion, Sydney, 1992

'Now I pray healing over you through the spirit of Jesus Christ our Lord. I pray for the Lord to bind the spirits of messy handwriting, emotional problems, homosexuality and other physical problems. In our Father's name, Amen!' The pastor was praying over me vehemently with all his might, his and the assistant's hands laid on me as well.

I sat there soaking the Holy Spirit in, fully filled with the utmost faith that miracles could and were about to happen to me!

He continued on: 'I have a prophecy or vision for you of the future … your handwriting will be a lot neater and you are married surrounded by children. You will be happy in your life …'

The praying continued and I nodded, saying, 'Amen! Thank you, God, thank you, God!'

After one or two hours of having my eyes closed, praying and concentrating, I blearily opened them, squinting at the light coming in. It felt like I had been walking through a strange fog of spiritual prayer warfare where there were supernatural consequences involved. The pastor, his assistant and I were so tired after such a long session, we all simply looked at each other with weary yet happy smiles on our faces. It was at that moment that I felt so close to my God, the Father in Heaven.

We walked outside to find my parents waiting and looking hopeful. The pastor said, 'With God's help we have done great work with Megan today. Amen to that!', and then he patted me on the back.

After several of these sessions it was concluded that I had been healed of my many afflictions, and all the evil spirits had been bound away. It was some type of prayer therapy—yet another form of the many therapies that we had tried in order to bring my life into some sort of balance over the years.

Healing, 2005

'Now, Megan. This healing weekend retreat conference will be of benefit to you and your Christian growth with God,' my adoptive mother for the weekend said, taking a firm grip on my arm. 'Don't worry. We will be there with you.' For a small woman she was full of physical as well as spiritual strength, a real warrior of God with such zeal.

So it was decided that I should go to a retreat conference to gain the benefits. On arrival we were welcomed before supper in the dining room. That evening the weekend of ministry began, then after supper we all toddled off to bed to rest before the full day ahead with its many different planned activities.

After the lights were turned off I had trouble sleeping and my mind was awash with anxiety. Different questions were going through my head about what to expect from the weekend and whether or if I would be healed.

The next day after breakfast the sessions continued on in full force until morning tea, then after that until lunch when a lot of people were chirpy about what was happening, including my adoptive parents for the weekend. We started talking about the weekend after lunch and how it was going for each of us. My adoptive mother then turned to me and said, 'Megan, by putting all their faith in God anyone can be healed, including you and your Asperger's condition. Megan, you can be healed. But you have to totally believe in it with all your heart, okay?'

She grabbed hold of me and gave me a firm squeeze of affirmation and support. What she had said was still sinking into my head and I didn't know whether to take it as helpful, well-meaning advice or an insult. I just agreed with her, but inside I felt a growing feeling of anger and confusion well up inside me for some unknown reason.

I needed to get away on my own for a bit and have a cigarette and a deep think. I got out a piece of paper and pen and started to write down questions and points for her to answer. Some of the questions were along the lines of, if someone is blind or deaf, can they be healed? Or if someone has cerebral palsy or Down syndrome, which physically affects their facial features and so forth, can they be healed totally from that? Or if someone was born with a congenital disability like Asperger's, then how can they be healed from that? What happens to the person involved when all the prayers of healing have been said and they are not healed? What happens to their belief in God after that?

I still had some more really curly questions to write down to ask her, but by this time she had beckoned me to come to the next session and I went along unwillingly. Not long into it I couldn't stand it any longer. I felt like bursting into tears and crying, so I walked out of the building. For some reason I didn't feel like worshipping and praying. Soon afterwards she followed me to see whether I was all right and at that point the floodgates burst along with questions and tears to match.

With all that I had to say I think the poor woman was rather taken aback and she went really quiet, which wasn't like her at all. She could see what I was saying and was left fumbling, trying to find words to explain everything. We agreed to disagree; I had felt it was important to stand up for myself and my condition.

I believe having Asperger's does not make me any less than anyone else in the sight of God, or that I am weaker as a result of that. Maybe it even proves I am stronger and tougher than the average person. I am who I am, no matter what happens!

Present Day

With all my different experiences of religion I have grown a lot in many different ways as a person. Sure I've been through a lot of times of doubt, questioning, confusion and saying that God was a Higher Power in 1996, when I was at one clinic.

Sure I do have a lot of questions about the way I am but I also accept that there must be a reason for it. I'm not claiming that I'm perfect and that I know the answers to things when I don't. Sometimes I don't go to church or Bible study every week but I feel I can miss a few here and there.

For me the most important part is having a personal relationship with God and I know within my heart that I am deeply committed and have come a very long way. I also know that if it were not for God and his guardian angels I'd be dead about eight times over! So I'm happy that he's looked after a person like me who's been a bit of a rogue but always had a heart.

Mum says when I get to heaven I will be able to recognise my guardian angel. He will be the tall one with bitten fingernails and most of his grey hair torn out!

The Mental Health System

The mental health system is extremely complicated. For some people in it, the support can grow into a habitual routine and they can become too reliant and institutionalised. They are often originally admitted during a crisis period to get support, then leave, have a relapse, go back in, see some people who were there the last time, go to groups, get into another routine—it becomes a very safe and familiar place, far away from the normal outside world. Sometimes it's almost too safe and it becomes a small community to which people keep returning for one reason or another.

As it turns out I was becoming one of those people who was getting way too dependent on the system and it was starting to wreak havoc in my life rather than helping me. I became desensitised to it and saw and experienced things that people on the outside wouldn't see or know about. I became 'in the know' of the secret lives of patients in clinics or hospitals.

I've never been to prison but I suppose in some ways it can be similar to a clinical environment where there are people trying to look after and monitor you. It's almost like being on the TV show *Big Brother*. Everyone is watching one another including the doctors and nurses who write in your file on an hourly basis. As a patient several times over in places like that, I have learned things both good and bad through the other patients.

You see a whole lot of different disturbed people from many types of backgrounds with every problem under this sunny sky of ours in those places. I've been in with Vietnam vets, WWII veterans, anorexics, bulimics, overeaters, people with bipolar disorder and multiple personality disorder, schizophrenics, psychotics, just to mention a few.

After a while you begin to think that you've got more than one thing wrong with you because you're hanging around other sick people, 24/7. That, believe it or not, has a huge impact on you and because of that you get a new social circle of understanding, caring and recovering 'friends'. I've heard stories that would make your skin crawl.

The secret goings-on of a lot of patients, with their dark hospital-type humour, can be pretty shocking to a newcomer to those places. There's almost a secret type of jargon and you're on a very steep learning curve about surviving in places like that.

It is easy sometimes to get lost in everybody else's problems and to forget your own. It's like a subculture where you can lose months, years or even decades of your life (and a lot of money also!) when you could've been doing better things. Sometimes people become stuck in a sort of mental health limbo for many years before they know it.

Some days I didn't know what was going to happen from one minute to the next because the situation was highly volatile with all the different patients and all of their different conditions. Those who have a few overlapping diagnoses are often the most sensitive to new and challenging events going on around them.

To be honest I don't know how the staff can deal with all the different stuff that the patients throw at them ... some literally! I know I could never do that type of work because it would be way too much and too close to home for me. I've had enough dramas in my life to last a lifetime ... so it's the quiet life for me all the way from now on.

So although over the years I fell into the crack that is the mental health system, the clinics and institutions have generally been good places to get help when I needed it. Because of the extremely dedicated staff, hundreds if not thousands of lives have been saved, including mine! But with the minimal government funding, more action has to be done to help educate more people about mental health issues.

11

Tricks Of The Trade—How I've Learned To Cope

Living with Asperger's is very confusing and tricky. It takes up a lot of emotional energy just dealing with the condition let alone trying to communicate with other people around you. When you walk into a room it's like a war zone, in a sense, with dozens of different signals, actions and gestures bombarding you in every direction. It is completely overwhelming to a person like me.

Yet over the years I have become better at trying to deal with different situations and also people. I'm not saying that I've got it completely right. It has taken a lot of hard work from me and also a lot of understanding from other people around me … mainly my family, also some friends.

Asperger's isn't a disease as I've heard some people call it. It also can't be healed or cured by God like a few of my Christian friends have said. It's not even a mental health issue as some other friends have told me. Asperger's is a simple syndrome that you were born with and came out of your mum's womb with.

Don't worry, because it isn't contagious and you can't catch it if you come too close to me. It doesn't mean that you are a freak if you've got it. It just means that you look at the world a little differently. You still have the same emotions and feelings as everybody else in this world. For me I've always had trouble understanding these emotions and how to express them in an appropriate way as an adult.

Often I've felt that I'm a child in an adult's body trying to understand the confusing world around me where everything is not black and white. It also hasn't got regimented rules, routines, patterns or structures where you can feel safe. Instead there are a lot of grey areas in what people say and do. Like they say one thing and then do something else and mean another thing again, which is in no way logical for me. Why can't people say what they really mean?

Living in this world for me has been like a massive freefall beyond belief with no parachute to save me. It's like trying to make up your own parachute by blowing up as many balloons as you can before you hit the ground rising up before you. Or maybe using feathers or branches and trying to flap your arms like wings as fast as you can to help you fly, yet still nothing is happening. You end up hitting the ground over and over emotionally, still trying to work out what went wrong—and trying to work out why you're different. You see a sky above you filled with parachutes having a great time doing their own thing, which you find very frustrating indeed. Your constant dream is of one day being able to fly with them, those people up in the sky, and being able to hold your own with them.

~

Here are some solutions—I call them 'tricks of the trade'—that I have picked up through trial and error. My family, doctor and friends have helped me learn these important life skills too.

When Someone Breaks Up With Me
- Don't do anything crazy, even when I feel like doing something.
- Don't call the person repeatedly, days or weeks after the break-up.

- If I do get to the point that I can't control myself with that, I should delete their numbers from my mobile phone, putting them on a different bit of paper so it's harder for me to get to.
- Try to let things be and accept what's happened in a grown-up manner, not letting my urges rule me.
- Try to feel and go with the emotions or grieving instead of fighting them or questioning them.
- Try not to forget that things will get better eventually!
- Try to put myself in the other person's shoes also.
- Pack up any gifts or things that remind me of the relationship, including photos. Put everything into a box or large plastic bag and then put that somewhere safe; don't look at them for quite a long time.

Trying To Relate Or Be Friends With People

- Listen properly to what they are saying.
- Give them a lot of space.
- Don't annoy them by contacting them all the time.
- Respect their opinions.
- Try to put myself in their shoes by being empathetic.
- Don't talk to them too much about myself, my problems and my life and remember to ask about their lives also.
- Don't ask too many questions—let people tell me things.
- Remember not to call anybody after 10.30pm or 11pm, unless it's a complete emergency.
- If I'm running late, call or text people to let them know what's going on.
- Very important: I don't have to tell them my life story overnight because they might freak out. Do it gradually!

When Meeting A Stranger

- Don't ask too many questions.
- Don't use any strange facial expressions or body language.

- Maintain eye contact and don't look around them or the room, getting distracted.
- Try to be well-mannered and not show my nerves too much towards the person.
- If someone has introduced me and is talking to someone else as well, try to include myself in the conversation instead of just standing there doing my own thing.
- Try not to judge too quickly when people are saying different things about themselves or their lives.
- Don't ignore them or fidget when they are around.
- Don't tell them my life story and all the information about myself because they may think I'm more than a bit strange.

Pub/Club Rules

Smoking:
- Always have an extra pack.
- If someone gives me a smoke, give it back the next time I light up.
- Always have enough cigarettes for an evening or a function.
- Always buy enough to replace what I have taken PLUS MORE.

Drinking:
- Never accept a drink unless I know people very well.
- Instead of drinking alcoholic drinks all night long, try to stagger it with one water and then one alcoholic beverage.
- Never leave my drink unattended, because it may get spiked.
- It is all right to have one or two drinks and say 'NO!' to the rest, even when other people are drinking around me.
- Never, ever get into a car with someone who's obviously been drinking a lot or drugging or is incapable of proper judgement, because I could end up in hospital or even killed.
- Always have some type of ID on me in case something happens. Important cards can be my driver's licence, pension card or healthcare card, Medicare card, bankcard if I need extra money, health fund card, or a piece of paper with my next of kin.

- Always have a bit of extra cash hidden somewhere in my wallet or on my person in case anything gets stolen.
- Don't ever leave the group that I have come with, or leave with a stranger or strangers because anything could happen to me.

Going To Parties

- If I'm asked to bring food, drink or something, take it along.
- Try to remember proper people-etiquette.
- If I'm lost or late, call or text them to let them know what's happening.
- See if I can help out with anything if I know the people really well.
- If kids or people get too much for me, go find a quiet space for five or 10 minutes to relax and do some deep breathing.
- If anxious, try not to look at my watch too much or when it's time to leave, because people could see that as a bit weird.
- Never leave before the birthday cake arrives because people might think I'm rude. So even when anxious, try to cope and stay.
- Don't walk off in the middle of conversations. Excuse myself and say what I'm doing so people are not left wondering.
- Try not to go off alone all the time or stand alone too much because people might think that a bit strange. Try to join in.
- Remember to try to take an interest in other people and ask them questions about themselves and their lives.
- Remember I can't apply the rules from one party to another exactly because each party, and the people there, are never the same. They are always different in really subtle ways. (This may also apply to friends and other people.)

Telephone Conversations

- Don't ring and then hang up the instant they answer because I'm too scared to talk to them. That might unnecessarily worry them.
- If I'm unsure of what to say beforehand, write the things down on

a bit of paper so I can remind myself during the conversation.

- Never hang up on people even though I might have had an argument and am angry with them.
- On the phone it is important to try to listen to people instead of interrupting them with what I want to say.
- Always listen and let a person finish what they are saying before I say my piece to them.
- Do not ever go suddenly dead silent on the phone because the person on the other end may think the line has gone dead or I am literally dead on my end.
- It's best not to do a monologue on the phone because the other person might get bored.
- Try not to 'Um!', 'Err!' or 'Ahh!' on the phone because that could get a bit too much for some people.
- Make sure there's no background noise on my end such as TVs, radios, CD-players, dishwashing machines, dryers, washing machines or other such appliances to distract people on the other end. They may find it hard to hear me.
- Talking loudly on the phone is not a good idea because I might deafen the other person. They are not on the other side of the room—only down the end of a phone line which is really quite close.
- Always call at appropriate times for the person and don't call past about 9:15pm at night or before 9am. Don't call during the night or in the early hours of the morning because the person won't be impressed. Only in emergencies can I call at strange times.

Staying Overnight

- Try to make sure I go to bed at the same time my hosts do out of courtesy.
- Try to remember to bring a torch with me for trying to find things at night-time.
- Also try to keep an eye out for things that need to be done in the

house that I can help with.

- Try not to stay more than two or three nights with the hosts because I may overstay my welcome without realising it.
- Always try to communicate and talk to my hosts about what is going on or if any problems have arisen.
- After I've stayed with them always try to send them a thank-you card or letter.
- If I'm going to be out late somewhere, always give them a call to let them know what's happening and that I'm okay.
- If the whole family and I go out for dinner, lunch or coffees, always pay my share adding a few dollars for incidentals such as tips.
- If they've lent me a front door key, always give it back to them at the end of the visit.
- While staying with my hosts, always accept their rules, boundaries, guidelines and beliefs. For example, if I'm not allowed to smoke inside or close to the house, go outside.

Dealing With Men Who Like Me More Than A Friend But I Don't Like Them Back

- Give very clear messages if I'm not interested in having a close relationship or friendship with him because it makes me feel uncomfortable. I am fine on my own, thanks very much!
- Try not to be alone with him.
- Do not invite him into my house reasonably late at night or visit him late at night, even if his flatmate is there.
- If he does help me out at all, thank him profusely or buy him a small gift of a couple of beers.
- If I do go out somewhere with a guy just as friends, don't let him pay. Always pay my own way because he could get the wrong message.
- Keep hugs at a bare minimum. Even if he asks for one, state my comfort level. If I feel comfortable, only give him a 'Hello' or 'Goodbye' hug or quick peck on the cheek.

- Don't ever go out and have one or more drinks with him, or get drunk, because he could take advantage of my inability to think properly with a lot of alcohol on board.
- Don't let him stay over in my house alone with me even if it's on the sofa bed in the lounge room, because anything could still happen.
- Always remember that all men might, and could have an ulterior motive with their actions towards me.
- Always remain very guarded until I get to know him really well, with time. That way his true colours will always start to show.
- Always apologise and say sorry if he feels I have led him on. Do say I'd always made it clear that all I wanted was friendship and nothing else.

Living Alone As a Woman

- Always lock doors and close all windows when going to bed at night.
- Before opening the door to someone who's knocked on it, always look through the peephole and ask 'who is it?'
- Don't leave any electrical appliances like dryers, dishwashers, washing machines on while I'm going out somewhere because it could catch fire or something. Or flood my home with water.
- When in the shower don't go running to answer the ringing phone because I could slip and hurt myself badly or even knock myself out. Always let it go to answering machine.
- Never invite strangers or people that I don't know well, or have only just met, back to my house late at night because I could be giving them the wrong message.
- Don't let people stay and sleep on my sofa bed until I've known them for a while and can trust them.
- At night always play my music low so my neighbours can't hear it or put headphones on instead. I don't want neighbours angrily trying to beat down my door.

- Don't try to be a 'fix it' woman around the house unless I definitely know what I am doing. If I don't know what to do hire a professional or get my good old reliable dad to do it.
- If in urgent need of help in the middle of the night and I can't reach my phone... Yell out 'Fire! There's a fire!' to let neighbours know something is wrong. It is a known fact that sometimes people may ignore you if you yell out 'Help!'
- Carry some type of personal alarm so people can hear me if I need them to.
- Make sure I are on speaking terms with a couple of trustworthy neighbours in case I ever need their help in a crisis.

12

Living As An Adult With Asperger's

W hile my love life was stumbling along through my 20s, my attempts at work and adult education also seemed cursed. All I had known when doing courses was that I had always seemed to fail badly!

After many years of not studying I found it so hard to adjust because the only form of structure I'd had was in clinics or support groups. Nothing really in the 'real world' at all. I would do reasonably all right until I started seeing someone who wasn't good for me emotionally.

One night in the middle of winter I went over to meet a date in Paddington and I heard a screech in the street and saw a dog hit and then run over by a car. I decided to cross the road to try to help. The dog, a Rhodesian Ridgeback mixed with something else, latched onto my hand.

It was still biting into my hand as I yelled out for others to help me and it took about three or four men to pry its jaws from my badly bitten hand. When they did I saw a huge puncture mark through it. My hand was so thin that the large tooth nearly went through my whole hand.

I rang my date, who arrived in time to see the aftermath. I nearly fainted because of the shock of it all. She drove my car to the nearby medical centre where a doctor cleaned the wounds, put in two stitches and gave me a tetanus shot for good measure. The doctor told us both to have a quiet night and a cup of tea to calm down.

As it happened, it was far from the quiet night the doctor ordered. Early in the morning my date decided to break it off with me after only a few weeks of seeing each other.

A couple of days after being bitten by the dog I ended up back at TAFE for my Basic Office Skills course with my badly damaged hand. I could hardly do any of the typing and other activities because of it, even though X-rays had revealed no broken bones, luckily. A week later I dropped out of the course because I had hardly any use of my hand.

~

AsI have mentioned, as a kid I never knew that I had Asperger's syndrome. I had been diagnosed with minimal brain dysfunction (MBD) and ADD, which is attention deficit disorder. I'd always had trouble concentrating on my schoolwork so I was put on Ritalin, which was the main drug of choice for the doctors treating ADD at the time. It helped for a bit but seemed to stop working after a while.

After I left high school I attempted several TAFE courses. The first was an Office Administration course, when I was 18, where I had a lot of hassles. I was so mixed up and out of my depth that I tried to kill myself and then eventually dropped out much to my own disappointment as well as that of my family.

Later I did a six-month hospitality course. The other people there were disabled—Down syndrome and intellectual disabilities—and much worse off than I was. I didn't like being there at all and it threatened me because at the time I hadn't been diagnosed with Asperger's, and had always believed I was not disabled.

But not all my study experiences ended in failure. The following year, in 1993, I did another six-month course in childcare at Randwick TAFE, run through the CES. I was living in Brookvale with my parents at the time and I was on crutches during most of that course because I'd had a mole removed from the sole of my foot. It was so annoying with very heavy bags getting on and off public transport. I also found and did the necessary work experience. The great bonus was that I found a job and worked for about a year as a childcare assistant, which I loved.

Unfortunately, then, my life took a turn for the worse and fell apart for a couple of years completely. I was admitted to a couple of clinics and found I had very little emotional energy left to further my education.

Trying to pull my life together, halfway through 1997 I did a Career Education Training for Women course through Seaforth TAFE that was run in association with the CES and Department of Social Security. At the time I was still getting over the abusive relationship that I had been in the previous year, so I was still in an extremely bad way emotionally. However, I managed to stick with the course, finding the required work experience, just happy to reach the end of it.

Early the next year I signed myself up to try to conquer the office administration course, which had got to me about seven years earlier. I was so determined to succeed with something that I had failed to finish before. At that point in time my family was dealing with a tough situation. My grandpa—the patriarch of my dad's family—was dying, which was very hard for us all. He died in late February.

Over the next few months I did end up falling out of the course again, although this time I approached the TAFE counsellor a few times for help. I remember being hugely disappointed that I had failed that course once again, but it did teach me the basics of typing, which I'm still using to this minute.

In the next few months the answers were coming regarding the mysteries of what was wrong with me. When I was diagnosed in 1998 with Asperger's syndrome it was a real turning point for me. Everything started slowly clicking into place; I understood what was happening to me and what had happened in the past. Having a firm diagnosis now meant that I could apply for a disability support pension.

Over the next few years I was still dealing with a whole lot of different issues and at one point in 2001 I had completely given up on my life in every way possible. I didn't want to be around anymore because I felt like I was a waste of space for everyone around me. During that time I was in and out of clinics because emotionally I was dead. Everything had finally caught up with me. I could see no future for myself.

After all this, in 2003 my doctor had the idea I should go to a specific place for educational help as well as work training. He recommended me to a place that mainly dealt with people with serious mental illnesses such as bipolar disorder, schizophrenia and all those types of conditions.

I've never been classified with a mental illness but to see other people around me with real mental problems was quite confronting and also a bit scary at times. I found myself smoking cigarettes again when I hung around with those people, which I felt bad about.

I felt that I was quite out of my depth, so didn't attend very often except for a part-time course with one of the best and most understanding teachers. She was teaching me one-on-one about computer and photocopying skills, which was really interesting. It was a do-it-at-your-own-speed type of course, which worked well for me.

We could go only when we felt able to participate and we made appointments once or twice a week, depending on how we felt. I ended up finishing the courses there and receiving two statements of attainment, which I felt so proud about. I hadn't received any type of certificate or anything like that for a long time. It felt great—quite amazing!

Partway through 2004 I decided to try to do a six-month course at Brookvale TAFE that didn't affect my pension. Yes, it was my third attempt at that bloody office skills course with one of the same teachers from one of the previous years when I tried it first off. To make it all worse, this was the 'dog-bite' course!

It was advertised through *The Manly Daily* for women wanting to brush-up their skills and get back to work in some form. The ladies were about my age or older and it was a smaller class, which was good for me. In the first few days I also fronted up to the Disability Learning Services at the college to finally sign up for help if I needed it. In the short time I was there, by all the teachers' accounts I was doing well with the course, but on the inside I was crapping myself.

Having Asperger's (and ADD) I have always found it hard to attend classes regularly and to finish things, even to persevere in some situations. Also I find some group dynamics quite confronting; they make me feel extremely anxious. I tend to isolate myself without asking for help, then quietly drop out.

I decided to do a course one day a week at TAFE. Most of the people in the course were more disadvantaged than me, younger than me, unable to drive, and still living at home with their parents. That day we all walked down to the cafeteria together where we had morning tea. I didn't talk much to the other students because I felt that I couldn't relate to them properly. Instead I found myself able to talk and interact with the teachers much better.

After that day I decided not to go back to that course. Instead I decided to do a part-time (one night a week) writing course run through a community college, which I had been given as a Christmas present from mum. Despite this I was still waiting to see what the Autism Society was doing with their course, which I thought was a much safer bet for me in the long term as far as employment went.

When I heard at last that the Autism Society's course had been scrapped for a variety of reasons, I felt so disappointed because I was really relying on them for help. After all, it is the only targeted avenue of help for people with Asperger's.

Since finding that out I did another part-time writing course for a few hours one day a week through the Manly Community College, which I finished in about May or June of that year. Then mum read about a memoir-writing course. It was only a few hours one day a week, which was good for me. I booked in and upon arriving at the centre on a Wednesday morning discovered that there was a group of about 12 to 15 of us. It was mostly older women, which I found interesting, with me being the youngster of the group. I remember feeling slightly awkward.

We started off with introductions, which was cool, then began doing easy writing exercises. Then, to my surprise, we had to read them out to the whole group, which I found difficult because I wasn't used to reading my work aloud.

Over the next few weeks I had a few teething problems but still kept on going because I thought that just turning up was an achievement in itself. It started getting easier as time wore on, yet I still had great trouble writing about personal things and sharing them with the group, with them listening to me. I thought that they would reject me and not accept me for myself because of what had happened to me in my life. In about October of 2005 the built-up stress all got to me and I had to go into a clinic for about a month.

I made sure that I got permission to attend the course during that time even though I had to catch public transport from the clinic, which I found confronting. That time was hard, but it was great to see everyone at the course each week. It made me feel more normal to be part of something outside the clinic. The course finished in December with a public event, reading our work to a gathering of our friends and families. It was very satisfying for me because I did finish the course right to the very end.

The next year there was an opportunity to go further with the course for one full year with the same teacher, who we all found very inspiring. During that year we were taught the basics of writing and also how to start to put together a book or memoir. It sounded great but was a bit expensive and too full-on for me, even though it was just a few hours each Wednesday.

As a Christmas present my parents decided to help pay for the course, and this meant so much to me. I was really scared because never before in my life had I completed or stayed with something for a whole year and still enjoyed it. Yet I was determined to at least give it a try to see whether I could do it. Some other ladies from the group were going to attend also, which made me feel more comfortable. So over the Christmas and summer holidays I tried to prepare myself for the trials of the coming year.

I realised that I had to try to turn up every week and let the teacher know if I was sick and couldn't make it. Also I couldn't escape from Sydney and do one of my long road trips to take my mind off what was happening.

On arriving back to the course in February I discovered that there were a few new faces added to the class, which was interesting. Now I had to get used to these new people and what they were like.

That year the group became really close and we learned a lot about one another as well as our writing abilities and styles. I met someone who inspired me enormously and we became best friends, kindred spirits if you will. Finally I had met someone who saw the real me. She accepted me and I accepted her as a person, which was great!

At the end of the year all of us had finished the course—including me—at last. I was so excited and happy because I'd actually completed a year-long course. This gave me great confidence in itself. All the other people in the group were happy for me too, because they knew how much it meant for me to keep going with it.

Although our teacher had moved away from Sydney, it was decided that the writing course would continue in 2007 with a weekly lesson emailed from her. She would also teach the same sort of course through the WEA in the city for a term on Thursdays. After the first term she planned to come back and teach the group.

So in the February I started going to both courses so that I could get the most out of them. I needed to do more writing for this book, which was now in progress. I was having relationship hassles that made it hard to keep going, but it was good to attend the courses because hearing other people's writing helped inspire me.

In term two, our teacher informed us she had work commitments overseas that she had to fulfil and she would return in about six months. So we sadly said a fond goodbye to her, wishing her every safe travel blessing on the way. It was decided among us ladies that we would keep the course going, but we'd split the responsibilities of taking the lesson.

Using the same format we were used to, every week someone would present the lesson that they had prepared themselves. So instead of students we were also learning to be teachers of the group in a sense, taking classes.

In October the group took a month's break. I went to Western Australia, my home state, for a holiday and also to do research for this book. Catching up with family and friends was a real memory-jogger of my early years. I also saw three of the towns and the houses that I lived in with my family years ago as a kid, which I felt I needed to do. It grounded me, somehow.

Near the end of October the group came back together for the last part of the year. Then it was decided to resume the course in February 2008, with a few smaller breaks rather than to coincide with school holidays—simply taking time out when one of us was sick, had commitments, or a planned trip. The group is still going, with fewer people, but is still as valuable as ever.

Through this writing course I feel that I have gained a group of surrogate mothers or aunties. Listening to all the wisdom and stories of all these older women has enriched me as a youngish woman.

I think each one of us has grown individually, as well as together. There is a real sense of friendship, sharing, care and camaraderie that we all look forward to every week.

I feel that, despite Asperger's and my various difficulties, I am continuing to climb this mountain of education and am conquering it each day, learning more about myself, as well as the important lessons of life.

13

Coming Out Of The Asperger's Fog

The Phoenix

A mighty and powerful bird
Rising from the ashes
Into a fiery luminous ball
Filled with vapoury life
Gliding through the sky
With the fury of a comet
But filled with great ease and strength
Soaring the whole universe
On the starlit nights
Bringing us through
To our own myths and fables.
As ordinary people
We look on this wonder
As sometimes a saviour
And relate to it
For we as people
Have come through the ashes

And out of the fire
To live again
Like the magical bird
The Phoenix.
But we forget sometimes
In our hearts
It's the Phoenix of life
Keeping us going
Into eternal learning
About ourselves
And other people.

© Megan Hammond, 1996

I wrote this many years ago during one of the worst patches in my life, when I didn't think I would survive, but it's relevant to everyone.

I wrote this poem, but look at me now! I am still here and I've risen out of the ashes like the mighty phoenix. Not by myself but with the help and support of many others around me over the years. After all, we're all in this together.

For too long I have lived with all the fear, shame and guilt of being supported by a government that didn't understand me or people like me. I'm of an older generation of people with Asperger's ... the past-it generation ... the misunderstood, experimental generation.

The younger generations of people diagnosed with Asperger's coming up around me have all the support and guidance that they'll ever need in their many years to come.

I was born in the wrong generation for the best help, but I feel that I have a massive responsibility to tell my story so that Asperger's can be understood and my life has counted for something.

Finally I am beginning to find my voice. Sometimes I was silenced by other people, but often I've been gagging myself. It turns out I have actually been stealing time from myself because of fear. For me that is a very big thing to realise, because that means I have to face the hard truth that it's all up to me. Sometimes I'm the hugest coward when things come to the crunch but my conscience and humanity always drive me to face up to the important things in life that really do matter.

In 2004, just after I came out of a clinic where I was receiving some therapy, I undertook the biggest part-time job of all. Inspired by my parents, I decided to start writing a book about my life and experiences with Asperger's syndrome. My aim was to try to help other people like me. So in fact I created the perfect type of job for me, doing something that I liked to do very much.

By going regularly to my writing course and making solid, unconditional friendships, I have gained an inner confidence. I do matter. I do have a voice not only to speak, but to shout and also sing so that others can hear me at last after all these years of silence!

Seeing my book slowly grow over the years has been an amazing experience. This book started to become full-time work and doing some work on it every day was challenging. I have found it rewarding to face up to my fears and relive my story. Over the past few years I have learned so much about going on with life. And I know this book of mine is written from the heart! It has been a huge job that I had to do for myself and for everyone out there who is living with Asperger's.

In the future I would like to see myself working in a job that is somehow helping others around me. Whether it is through writing, speaking or some other hidden talent that I am yet to discover.

The Asperger's fog has lifted and life is a whole lot clearer, but the future is a mystery. I'll just have to wait and see what happens …

14

Notes From Megan's Family

Megan's Mum's Story

Years ago, before I was married, I taught for a while in 'special schools'. While the children had a range of disabilities, I remember one boy in particular who had autism. He was totally removed from the world of his fellow classmates, and would spend the day walking up and down the steps of his classroom. Up and back, up and back, hooting occasionally.

So I knew, absolutely, that Megan, our long-awaited, much cherished first child did not have autism. She was friendly and outgoing for starters. Okay, perhaps a little too outgoing, but we had a wide circle of friends and people dropped in often, so she had more than enough opportunity to become sociable.

She was, though, 'different' in other ways. Even as a new baby she slept very little, preferring to lie quietly in her cot. As she grew older she played quietly on her own too—her younger brother didn't arrive until she was aged two years and seven months—absorbed for hours, it seemed, lining up her toy animals and blocks in rows.

Although her speech was delayed, she had her own language in which she was most fluent. She must have imagined that there was something wrong with these parents of hers who could not even understand her simplest sentences. She had an incredible memory too and could locate things we had misplaced around the house and, as her language baffled us more and more, she found a way of communicating, flicking quickly through one of her many books until she found a picture of whatever it was she was trying to tell us about. Aha! At four years old that 'gargahoo' she had been almost crying in frustration about appeared in the story of Noah's Ark. There it was—a *kangaroo*—lined up ready to survive the flood.

All the 'milestones' of babyhood were more or less ticked off—teeth popped through on time, a first 'mum, mum' (or so it sounded to these immensely proud, unskilled parents), crawling (okay, a bit slide-on-the-stomach, but propulsion anyway), standing and then walking by 15 months. Nothing too much to worry about, surely.

Yet the concern remained—call it a mother's niggling premonition, if you like. In fact we both sensed something was not quite right. We had many nights before sleeping where we went through the options: her hearing is fine, her sight is excellent. She understands what we say to her and can find something we ask for or do something she is asked to do, so she can't be intellectually disabled, can she? Is she autistic? No, she is too friendly, too loving, too with us.

Sure, she had funny little ways, but many children do as they try on different behaviours, and she wasn't a naughty child. There was a just a 'can't-put-my-finger-on-it' something that had us concerned enough to take her to a few doctors who patted our hands and in effect said 'there, there, she'll grow out of it', which is what we wanted to hear and had half-expected anyway.

As an ex-school teacher, I had some early childhood IQ tests somewhere so when she was about five years old I tested her and she came out well above normal. Well, that was a relief!

Megan's childhood passed with the usual sibling rivalry and conflict, but her understanding of discipline and her limited concept of cause and effect became markedly obvious as her brother, Cameron, grew and developed. I quickly found that I needed to reason with and discipline them quite differently as her needs became more apparent. So often it seemed she had to actually experience something for her to realise its danger or importance. In one of our late-night Megan-discussions, we finally agreed that cognition was at the core of her problem.

She would become obsessed with things and people, too, and seemed totally unable to move from her position if she wanted to do something. Her behaviour as a young child was often inappropriate—dancing on the lawn in a singlet in winter or refusing to take off a jumper on a scorching 40°C summer day in Geraldton, Western Australia both come to mind. In fact her ability to not know whether it was hot or cold was a mystery to us. For many years she would ask, 'Is it a hot day today?'

Even more worrying were the bizarre things—tying naked Barbie dolls to sticks in the garden, or filling her school case with rocks and leaves on the way home from school and then spreading them under her bed. It was like a park under there!

Megan would also get what we called her 'black look', which turned her lovely brown eyes into flat inky pools of resistance. We sensed that nothing—certainly no punishment—could ever make her back down from her position. I plumbed the very depths of my creativity to find a way that we could still keep our position without breaking her spirit or (worse) losing our own self-control.

One of the hardest things when you have an 'unusual' child is to know how much is a childhood phase, how much is pure genetics— my husband Gordon and I have 'quirky', creative (okay, a few eccentric) people in both our family trees—and the question becomes, how much 'difference' is something to worry about and deal with? No parent wants to make a child more aware of any 'problems' they may have, yet we felt it would be a tragedy if there was something we should be addressing early, that might spare her problems in the future.

So began a round of doctors, specialists and therapists. There were various diagnoses: minimal brain dysfunction and ADD the only ones with a name, but no therapy, tablet or exercises seemed to provide what we were looking for—a magic bullet to fix whatever it was.

Megan has dealt with all of this in the rest of this book. For us it was a time of repressed concern as we continued to treat her as a normal average child. We refused to say she had a disability or to deal with her in any way other than normal. She was loved equally, obeyed the same family rules her brother did (even if they were a bit of a mystery to her sometimes) and attended a mainstream school and perplexed her teachers as much as she did us.

Perhaps this is the most difficult aspect of what we now know she was affected by—Asperger's syndrome. On the one hand Megan was a bright, intelligent, attractive child and teenager. 'There's nothing wrong with her,' is a comment we have heard so often; 'She looks absolutely normal.' And she does, but it was a backhanded insult, really, which often left us feeling that maybe we were the only difficulty Megan had.

Were we actually creating a monster—a child with severe psychological problems—because we were trying to uncover some mythical point of difference? Was it us who were simply turning her into something else? It was an unspoken guilt that had us searching our consciences more than once.

The teenage years were turbulent—but then aren't they often for any youngster? Somewhere I have read that most teenagers have a clinical form of Asperger's syndrome as their hormones and brain chemistry ebb and flow. Who knows? Certainly the elements of reckless risk-taking, lack of understanding of other people's points of view and scrambled cognition are similar. Let's just say that adolescence and Asperger's is a tough mix.

It took 26 years for us to learn that there was a name for the root of all Gordon's and my concerns and, by then, Megan's immense sadness and frustration. Today's youngsters are assessed and diagnosed correctly so much earlier. Their parents at least have a diagnosis and can get on with the business of dealing with Asperger's, which is all we ever wanted do anyway, of course. The children, too, have the relief of understanding that they are not lazy or stupid or geekish, or whatever tag society might be prepared to put on them.

In Megan's case we learned that she had an additional diagnosis of ADD (which is not unusual we have been told) but without the hyperactivity. Hers is *hypo*-activity, which is in its own way just as challenging as Asperger's. I describe it by saying she has difficulty finding and activating her 'on' switch in order to access the energy and enthusiasm we all need to begin a task or continue it for any length of time.

Perhaps this is why, on two levels, I am immensely proud of Megan for finishing this book. Not only has she diligently applied herself to telling her story and writing many thousands of words, but by doing so she has been incredibly honest and open in sharing some highly personal parts of her life. She has done it, in her words, 'to help others understand Asperger's'.

As a mother—as Megan's mother—I would like other parents to know that while Asperger's is a real and major challenge for families and individuals, there can be hope and triumph too. Megan has shown, against enormous odds, that this is so.

Sally Hammond

Megan's Dad's Story

'If you're happy and you know it, clap your hands!'
I can still see Megan singing this song as a child with great enthusiasm, flapping hands and out-of-sync claps. Music has always been one of the joys of her life, even if rhythm has not been her greatest strength. Here a couple of other variations of the same little song:
If you're different and you don't know it,
You don't care!
And then there is Megan's version:
If you are different and you know it, and others know it,
Shit begins.

Human beings generally don't do 'different' very well. It might seem strange when you consider that the part of the paradox of understanding human behaviour is found in resolving the tension of how we are amazingly similar yet so incredibly dissimilar. You'd think that we should have a handle on it by now, but as a society we have a long way to go. We go over the top with positive difference. Just look at the excessive manner in which celebrities are glorified. But we shun and run when it comes to any negative deviation from the norm.

It is the platform of comedy and jokes. Did you hear the one about the Irishman, the Scotsman and the Australian? One way of dealing with and disguising the discomfort of difference is to laugh at it. Just ask Megan.

It is a major cause of prejudice. People from other countries, who speak another language, who believe in another God, whose physical appearance doesn't match ours, are not welcome, especially if they arrive in a water-logged fishing boat. We don't mind visiting them in their own countries but do we really want them in our backyard? They are okay as long as we can maintain that distance. It hurts like hell to see your daughter become the butt of jokes and experience endless rejection because she is what I often describe as 'almost normal'.

What happens when a child is born 'different'. When I first held Megan in my arms, only minutes after her birth, there was nothing to suggest that she was anything other than a normal infant. She passed all the mandatory tests. The little bits and pieces were perfectly formed. I couldn't have been a happier and prouder father. But, as any parent knows, the journey only begins at birth and bringing up a child is full of surprises. We had our share waiting for us. It wasn't too long before we started to ask some serious questions. We couldn't put a finger on it and it would take many years before we could put a name to it. It niggled and it was unsettling. Were we overreacting? Was there something we should be doing? Was there any form of professional help that could enlighten us? We really had no idea what we were contending with.

In many ways she was just a normal kid with a speech defect. Other people generally didn't pick up on her unusual ways. Kids develop at different rates and Megan came across as a quiet little girl who didn't say very much. She was gregarious and often overly demonstrative, but developed her own unique ways of relating to others.

When I look back over her first 10 years I see many smiles and hear lots of laughter. Megan wasn't a bad kid. She could be difficult at times, incredibly stubborn and intransigent with some strange and often bizarre habits. We provided a tremendous amount of stimulus for her with plenty of physical activity, swimming, riding her bike, going for walks, playing rough and tumble games. She was much loved, bright and obviously intelligent. And the strange ways? Well, we did what any parent would do. We focused on them with ample diligence to lessen their impact and their apparentness. She was almost normal and we received repeated assurances that she would eventually grow out of it, whatever 'it' was.

Today it is almost becoming a fad to diagnose many behavioural problems as ADHD, or ADD or Asperger's. Sometimes I think we should begin with a good look at the diet of the family, time spent watching TV and playing video games, parenting practices and other glaringly obvious factors. Are we at risk of taking the easy diagnostic option? Who knows? Maybe the incidence of Asperger's is on the rise and we are witnessing the impact of years of using plastics, hydrocarbons, toxins and pollutants which are tampering with the genetic make-up of more and more children. Maybe it has always been around and we simply had no mechanism to diagnose it. One thing is certain. If your child has Asperger's, there is no doubting it. Certainly take every advantage of early intervention, but don't necessarily expect it to go away. It is something you learn to live with, not cure. It does help to know what you are dealing with. I felt like we were boxing blindfolded for 25 years.

There is a certain irony in me saying this. Over time I began to resent the implication that Megan's problems began with the home environment. The fact is that we knew we had a child with a special need and were committed to ensuring that the foundations for effective parenting were in place while we addressed her specific developmental issues. Discipline was firm but fair. Boundaries were clearly established and maintained. She was not punished or penalised because she was unusual. We worked as a team and made decisions jointly. On the other hand she received few concessions or preferential treatment. She grew up in a very loving and stable home, something which I think she finally recognises and appreciates as an adult. There are probably things we would do differently now in hindsight, but we were doing it on our own back then. Whether by good luck or by good management, we used many of the strategies that are now part and parcel of the clinical response to Asperger's. Our home has always been a very safe place, and today it is still a retreat for Megan when it all becomes too hard.

The older she became, the steeper the mountain we seemed to be climbing. More and more external influences began to accentuate the negative and eliminate the positive. This began to impact seriously on our ability to parent her. Peers were the quickest to spot differences and the most ruthless in capitalising on them. During adolescence others effectively countered every move we made to stabilise a disturbed life. Teachers were a mixed bag, with some going to great efforts to try and understand (dear sweet, patient, understanding Mrs Brighteyes), while others were as cruel as the kids. Maybe they figured that they were paid to teach, not solve the compounded behavioural quirkiness of a problem child.

Ironically, many of the professionals seemed to be the slowest to recognise just how different Megan was. Maybe it had to do with their training and the discipline of relying on methodology and procedure. Many seemed to look for answers in psychological models. The problem was that when Megan was a child there was no model and no label that fitted. They tended to rely on models that correlated behavioural problems with dysfunctional families. I have lost count of the number of professionals who began with the conclusion that there was nothing unusual or wrong with the child. The inference was obvious. Most eventually handed the problem back to us, acknowledging that there was indeed a problem, but the solution was not in the realm of their speciality. I almost came unstuck when the family was referred to Sydney's top adolescent and family counselling unit.

After an hour of very frank and transparent self-disclosure on our part, they apparently came to conclusion that I was abusing Megan in some way, probably sexually. I don't think I have ever felt so vulnerable or been so angry. It was a classic damned if you say something and damned if you don't situation, which could have seen the family split by the courts. Fortunately, with nothing to hide and a background in psychology, counselling and pastoral care which gave me professional equity, I confronted the team with their incompetence. They had completely disregarded the recognised protocols for cases of suspected abuse which exist to protect both children and parents. That clinical relationship was terminated very quickly.

Over the years we experienced the usual tensions found in parent–child relationships. We anticipated the transitions and accepted that things would probably be tougher to deal with as she reached puberty. The mixed bag of hormones, adolescence, identity, relationships, school, the desire for independence, loud music, messy room, defiance, rudeness, laziness, boyfriends, girlfriends … get my drift! They were all to be expected, and we were not disappointed. Asperger's compounded everything.

From about10 years of age Megan detached herself emotionally from me. It was irrational, confusing and often hurtful. I am still not entirely sure what triggered it, but if I so much as brushed past her she would scream and shout and perform 'something awful'. I couldn't come near her. It may have had to do with the fact that she blamed me for removing the family from her happy, secure world in Western Australia to a life of teasing hell in Sydney. For the first time in her life she was really confronted with her difference. She was tormented endlessly by the kids while the teacher watched it all happen. It was here that she entered the sad, confused world of the victim. It took the best part of 10 years before the barriers began to lift. She couldn't enunciate or identify what was going on, and we couldn't get to the bottom of it. That's Asperger's for you. You learn to accept it and work your way through and around it. It was during this period that we approached the adolescent team I referred to earlier.

The tide finally turned forever on the night that I turned up on her doorstep with a removal van and physically rescued her from a frighteningly abusive domestic relationship with Suzie. Sally was overseas and Megan was without her reliable emotional backstop. She was alone and devastated. It began to dawn on her that I really did love her and that I would stand by her come hell or high water. Maybe dad was okay after all. She was a mess and needed all the support I could give her. I suspect that, for the first time, she twigged that relating to me was quite different to the way she relates to her mother. Up till then I suspect that she only saw me as dad, not as a person.

I would not like to revisit those years for her sake as well as mine. We have forged a warm, affectionate relationship now. I recognise a level of sensitivity, intelligence and determination to succeed that I hadn't seen earlier. I am much closer to seeing the real person than I have ever been. She has made great strides in recent years and I think that she has the potential to extend herself even more. How this happens remains to be seen. I would like to see her enjoying greater financial independence though. Few things are more invalidating or disempowering than a living off a meagre pension. Like many parents whose children fall through the cracks we continue to support Megan in many material ways while receiving no benefits or tax relief. The financial cost is substantial, but we don't begrudge a cent of it and we wouldn't have it any other way. It is a small price to pay for her independence and our peace of mind. She does have a reasonable quality of life, is remarkably thrifty and manages her affairs well.

I don't think that we stand out as being exceptional parents. Like many who find themselves with a different child, we have risen to the occasion and often surprised ourselves by doing exceptional things. We certainly made our share of mistakes and much of the time were left to invent our own rules. I would be surprised if my years as an Adventist minister would have had much of a negative impact. I had left denominational employment by the time Megan was in her teens so she was not under any pressure to conform to the rather straight up and down rules of the church. On the contrary, her formative years provided a loving and moral foundation which is all too sadly lacking in many homes today. Even the damage perpetrated by church schools had more to do with incompetent individual teachers than the worthy principles of Christian education. Ultimately she has made her own faith and belief choices, which is the way it should be.

For me, the hardest thing was that we felt very alone. No-one else really understood, and worse still, many misunderstood. Professionals so often came to the wrong conclusion. It was terribly distressing watching her being admitted to clinics treating addiction, bipolar disorders, anorexia, schizophrenia and other forms of mental illness. I really do not think that Asperger's is a mental illness. Rather it is a cognitive and emotional dysfunction. The most enduring result of these admissions was the relationships she formed with other clients who compounded her problem. There was, and still is, no proper therapeutic context for Asperger's. I have the greatest respect for the doctors and staff who stood by her. Without their intervention I think the battle would have been lost. But they were not equipped therapeutically for the challenges that she presented.

There was no respite. Immediate family felt sorry us but never became involved. She baffled them. Finally, when her syndrome was at last diagnosed, I found it healing to see the pieces of the puzzle fall into their right places. The resolution meant that at last we understood and were understood, no longer alone. Mind you, for all the advances that have been made in understanding Asperger's, very little is happening for adults with the condition. They still fall through the cracks.

Megan's daily challenge is the same issue we faced for many years— that of being understood. Few take the trouble to discover the core person. There is a real person. Emotional handicap is probably the unkindest handicap. Megan experiences the full gamut of emotions as intensely as anyone else, but she lacks the cognitive circuitry to know how to respond to situations that most people learn intuitively. Imagine what it is like to experience emotions without understanding why they arise and not knowing how to respond to them. Welcome to Asperger's world. Every response has to be laboriously learned. She is one gutsy lady who has fallen in the shit many times, but keeps getting up and trying again. I admire her tenacity and am one proud father.

We both find great inspiration in the Serenity Prayer.

'God grant me the serenity to accept the things I cannot change,

The courage to change the things I can

And the wisdom to know the difference.'

Gordon Hammond

The Little Brother's Story

I am Cameron, the 'little brother' of Megan (aka Megs to me). I will try to explain a little bit about how Megan's Asperger's has affected me as well as my observations about how it's affected her.

Life as young kids was seemingly normal We were like any other brother and sister exploring the world together. We would do all the usual things that brothers and sisters do, playing games, fighting about who would get choice of a television show, eating ant sandwiches, the usual stuff.

But Megan was always a little bit different and I didn't know why.

I think the first time I remember noticing anything wrong with Megan was her chin-cup. The chin-cup was black and leather and looked like a slingshot that would fit around her chin and fasten behind her head. Megan would wear the chin-cup at night-time while she slept. Mum and dad explained that the chin-cup was part of Megan's 'speech therapy'. It was one of many attempted speech correction methods. I remember visiting speech therapists often. It was a common family outing.

Even though Megan is $2^{1}/_{2}$ years older than I am, it didn't take long for me to equal and then surpass her level of speech proficiency. I guess speech is one of the most obvious things that kids pick up on when establishing another kid is different. Unfortunately kids don't use words as sensitive as 'different' when announcing their discoveries. Teasing is one of the worst traits of human behaviour and Megan's subtle differences attracted more than her fair share of teasing.

While I'm on the topic of Megan's teasing, I need to mention some of the guilt I feel as a result of my childish actions, not as a self-indulgent way of making myself feel better but to hopefully help others to be more understanding than I was and avoid hurting people they care about.

Although we lived together harmoniously most of the time, I still feel a lot of guilt from all the times I teased my sister. Kids tease their brothers and sisters all the time but sometimes it's just not a fair match.

Megan never stood a chance; she may have been older than me but I had the artillery to win a word battle with ease. I knew it wasn't sporting, I knew it was wrong, but I did it anyway. I think the main reason was frustration, it made me angry trying to communicate with Megan, I was angry because she wasn't normal.

Many traits associated with Asperger's are frustrating for the people who they are close to. I'm talking about things like selfishness, tantrums, stubborn behaviour, even basic communication can be extremely frustrating when dealing with somebody with this condition. I hope that now being able to identify some of these behaviours early will mean parents can explain the condition to their kids before they use teasing as a retaliation to their sibling's frustrating behaviour.

Something I used to find most frustrating was Megan's stubbornness! When Megan decided 'no!' there was no amount of logical, rational discussion that could change her mind. This would frustrate me no end as I was also stubborn by nature and was always ready to argue until my case was won. But you can't hold a debate with someone who refuses to talk or even move ... indefinitely!!

The stubbornness would often escalate to tantrums, which I found impossible to deal with because there is just no way to communicate with somebody mid-tantrum. How ironic that I was frustrated about communicating with Megs when in hindsight it's so obvious that these tantrums stemmed from Megan being frustrated by her inability to communicate.

In a lot of ways Megan's disability made things easy for me, she made me look good.

Here's an example. I was eight and Megan was 10 and the time was approaching to move into a new house. Mum and dad, being the even-handed diplomatic types, had decided the fairest way to settle which child got the first choice of new bedroom was to have a 'keeping room clean competition'. No prizes for guessing who got the big room. Megan never had a chance of making the judgements she needed to keep ahead of me, even when the competition had rules as simple as cleaning up a mess.

I just remember thinking how easy this was for me. It was like taking candy from a baby. And as I kid I didn't care, I had a bedroom with a balcony. The older child ended up with a skylight! I think the whole family thought Megan would learn from these losses but it didn't seem to work. Megan never beat me at one of these supposedly even competitions. This must've been very frustrating for her.

Looking good had its downsides, though.

On one hand the differences between Megan and me made me look good, made me stand out, but … along with looking good came pressures and expectations that weren't always easy to deal with. They would normally be things mum and dad would say like 'We expect more from you' or 'you have no excuses'. Well, in my opinion just being an adolescent was an excuse. This was hard for me. I sometimes felt like I had to keep my parents doubly happy to compensate for Megan's shortcomings. But mum and dad are right and you should consider yourself lucky when other people are dealing with a lot—but try telling that to a self-absorbed rebellious teenager.

Finally, a moment of clarity.

I came to what I consider to be a real point of understanding about eight or so years ago. Something hit me really hard and has stayed with me ever since. By this time Megan had been diagnosed as having Asperger's syndrome and was consequently eligible for the government's disability pension. What a positive thing for Megs, some financial assistance and less pressure to be regularly employed.

I remember asking mum why Megs was taking so long to go to the Centrelink office to process the forms that would start the weekly payments? Traditionally it's laziness that stands in her way, but it wasn't like Megs to be lazy when it came to free money. When mum told me the reason was that Megan was embarrassed about being disabled, my stomach sank! This was my epiphany; this is when I realised how frustratingly close she was to being normal … normal enough to not only know she was different but also so close that she is embarrassed about it. This broke my heart! It said so much to me about what she has had to deal with through her life … how life must be for someone who is so close to normal, but different enough to make so many of the things we take for granted so challenging.

I guess I'd always hoped that part of her disability meant things weren't as painful for her. I mean, in the way a Down syndrome person is always so happy, seemingly oblivious to their differences. Sometimes I've wondered if being 'more disabled' would be better than 'being nearly normal ... but not quite'.

In recent years our relationship has become a bit like I am the older brother/life coach who dishes out advice with discerning bluntness. Maybe my hardline approach stems from 34 years of accumulated angst or maybe just because it seems to work. She seems to really respect and listen to my opinions and I'm sure she has the best intentions of following my orders, although her lack of motivation still ensures I don't run out of things to demand.

Even though I act like a tough talking sports trainer who is disappointed in a result, the reality is I am probably more like a frustrated coach who is just trying to keep motivation levels high and boost morale.

The truth is I am amazed at how far Megs has come and I admire the way she has bounced back from repeated failed relationships and serious bouts of depression.

The courage and endurance she has shown throughout her life is a testament to her character. I am not as strong nor as capable of handling traumatic experiences as Megan. Any hardships I have ever had to face are minuscule compared to what I have witnessed my sister endure! I take my hat off to her. I might be too proud to say it very often but I really respect Megan and I am a very proud little brother.

Cameron Hammond

Appendix

Autism Spectrum Australia

Autism spectrum disorders (ASDs) are lifelong developmental disabilities characterised by marked difficulties in social interaction, impaired communication, restricted and repetitive interests and behaviours and sensory sensitivities. The word 'spectrum' is used because the range and severity of the difficulties people with an ASD experience can vary widely. ASDs include autistic disorder, Asperger's syndrome and pervasive developmental disorder—not otherwise stated, which is also known as atypical autism. Sometimes the word 'autism' is used to refer to all ASDs.

Studies show that one in 160 Australians have an ASD and that it is more prevalent in boys than girls. The effects of an ASD can often be minimised by early diagnosis and with the right interventions, many children and adults with an ASD show marked improvements.

The three main areas of difficulty are:

1. Impairment in social interaction, which may include limited use and understanding of non-verbal communication such as eye gaze, facial expression and gesture, difficulties forming and sustaining friendships, lack of seeking to share enjoyment, interest and activities with other people and difficulties with social and emotional responsiveness.

2. Impairment in communication, which may include delayed language development, difficulties initiating and sustaining conversations, stereotyped and repetitive use of language such as repeating phrases from television and limited imaginative or make-believe play.

3. Restricted and repetitive interests, activities and behaviours, which may include unusually intense or focused interests, stereotyped and repetitive body movements such as hand flapping and spinning,

repetitive use of objects such as repeatedly flicking a doll's eyes or lining up toys, and adherence to non-functional routines such as insisting on travelling the same route home each day.

In addition to these main areas of difficulties, individuals with an ASD may also have unusual sensory interests such as sniffing objects or staring intently at moving objects, sensory sensitivities including avoidance of everyday sounds and textures such as hair dryers, vacuum cleaners and sand and intellectual impairment or learning difficulties.

The term ASD is an umbrella description which refers to three different diagnoses. Regardless of the specific diagnosis given, individuals with an ASD will experience difficulties in many different social situations such as school and work.

Autistic disorder (sometimes referred to as classic autism)
The diagnosis of autistic disorder is given to individuals with impairments in social interaction and communication as well as restricted and repetitive interests, activities and behaviours that are generally evident prior to three years of age.

Asperger's disorder (often referred to as Asperger's syndrome)
Individuals with Asperger's disorder have difficulties with social interaction and social communication as well as restricted and repetitive interests, activities and behaviours. They do not have a significant delay in early language acquisition and there is no significant delay in cognitive abilities or self-help skills. Asperger's is often detected later than autistic disorder as speech usually develops at the expected age.

Pervasive Developmental Disorder–Not Otherwise Specified (PDD-NOS sometimes referred to as atypical autism)
The diagnosis of PDD-NOS or atypical autism is made when an individual has a marked social impairment but fails to meet full criteria for either autistic disorder or Asperger's disorder. These individuals may also have communication impairments and/or restricted and repetitive interests, activities and behaviours.

ASD is diagnosed through an assessment which includes observing and meeting with the individual, their family and service providers. Information is gathered on the individual's strengths and difficulties, particularly in the areas of social interaction and communication as well as repetitive interests, activities and behaviours.

Such information may be obtained by administering standardised tests or questionnaires. ASD is usually diagnosed in early childhood, but assessments can be undertaken at any age. There is no single behaviour that indicates ASD. There are no blood tests that can detect ASD. If you have concerns, your GP may refer you to a developmental paediatrician or diagnostic assessment service in your area. Alternatively, you may contact Autism Spectrum Australia (Aspect) on 02 8977 8300 about the Aspect Diagnostic Assessment Service.

Currently, there is no single known cause for ASD, however recent research has identified strong genetic links. ASD is not caused by an individual's upbringing or their social circumstances. There is presently no known cure for ASD. However, early intervention, specialised education and structured support can help develop an individual's skills. Every individual with ASD will make progress, although that will depend on a number of factors including the unique make-up of the individual and the type and intensity of intervention. With the support of family, friends and service providers, individuals with ASD can achieve a good quality of life.

Aspect

Autism Spectrum Australia (Aspect) is Australia's largest not-for-profit autism specific service provider. Aspect builds confidence and capacity in people with an autism spectrum disorder (ASD), their families and communities by providing information, education and other services. Established in 1966, Aspect's specialised evidence-based autism educational program incorporates:
• Direct services for children in the form of early intervention and schooling, incorporating six specialty schools, over 70 satellite

classes, education and family support, assessment and transition and itinerant education support

• Direct services for adults in the form of employment, training and accommodation

• Advice and assistance for many families who are either receiving inadequate or inappropriate services, or for whom there are no services at all

• A central resource for families and services seeking information and advice about autism spectrum disorders, including Asperger's syndrome in NSW.

Aspect employs highly skilled professionals who are experts in the field of autism and who provide programs that emphasise the development of communication skills, social skills and independent living skills. The overall objective is integration into mainstream education, which in turn overcomes a major barrier to community living for people with autism.

Aspect offers a free service called the Aspect Autism Information Line, for people across Australia who have an ASD, as well as for their families, carers, support staff and professionals. It is staffed by professionals from a number of disciplines, and has available a wide range of information about services and resources.

Phone: 1800 069 978 (NSW only) or 02 8977 8377 between 9am and 4pm on weekdays. If staff are busy on other calls, please leave a voice message, and your call will be returned at the first opportunity.

ASPIA

Over the past decade there has been an upsurge of awareness and diagnosis of autism and Asperger's syndrome. Most of the cases being identified are children. For adults with Asperger's syndrome, their behaviour since childhood has gone underground and layers of coping strategies and defence mechanisms greet the social world. These behaviours often give the impression of someone quite together—perhaps a little eccentric or odd—but passable because of their high intelligence, impressive knowledge, high integrity and particular flair or gift in an area or career. Many adults with Asperger's syndrome marry and have children. However the experience of the partners and children are quite different to what most partners would experience and expect. Partners of an adult with Asperger's syndrome often have awareness early in the marriage that something is not right but they can't work out what.

Asperger Syndrome Partner Information Australia provides information on how Asperger's syndrome impacts on adult relationships and what steps can be taken to reduce the confusion, conflict and crushing emotional experiences that characterise the lives of those affected. They organise monthly support group meetings and seminars and promote awareness about the condition. They also produce a monthly newsletter. They are based in New South Wales but their website has links to other related groups throughout Australia. They also publish a list of professionals specialising in this area.

Further Information

Asperger Syndrome Partner Information Australia
http://www.aspia.org.au
Autism Spectrum Australia
www.autismspectrum.org.au
Autism New Zealand Inc
http://www.autismnz.org.nz
Autism South Africa
http://www.autismsouthafrica.org
Asperger's Syndrome Foundation (UK)
http://www.aspergerfoundation.org.uk
US Autism & Asperger Association (USAAA)
http://www.usautism.org